Behind the Consultation
Reflective stories from clinical practice

Andre Matalon, MD
and
Stanley Rabin, PhD

Forewords by
Benyamin Maoz
and
John Salinsky

Radcliffe Publishing
Oxford • New York

Radcliffe Publishing Ltd
18 Marcham Road
Abingdon
Oxon OX14 1AA
United Kingdom

www.radcliffe-oxford.com
Electronic catalogue and worldwide online ordering facility.

British Library Cataloguing in Publication Data

A catalogue record for this book is available from the British Library.

ISBN-13 978 1 84619 205 0

Typeset by Egan Reid, Auckland, New Zealand
Printed and bound by TJI Digital, Padstow, Cornwall, UK

Behind the Consultation

Reflective stories from clinical practice

Contents

Foreword

Two therapists, a clinical psychologist (Stanley Rabin) and a family physician (Andre Matalon), wrote these case narratives to each other over a long period of time. The narratives describe episodes in their relationships with patients that left a mark upon the therapists, often continuing to echo in their memory.

After years of maintaining this unique personal and professional, at times very intimate correspondence they decided to publish these dialogues, for professionals, as well as for the broader, interested public. This decision, too, was accompanied by the questioning that is at the heart of this book – why is there a need, or even a desire, to tell and to write stories from medical and psychotherapeutic practice to a colleague and then to publish them?

I shall try to relate to some aspects of this question.

"It is not good that man should be alone" (Gen., 2, 18) – the need for a mate was clear even in the Garden of Eden, and is doubly clear here on earth, where therapists and family physicians work very much alone. During the workday they might have an opportunity to walk into a colleague's room and tell of something that happened "just now" with a patient, but such encounters are occasional and informal. Therapists and physicians are human, and as such, it is not good that they are alone. They need a person to whom they can talk spontaneously about what happened with a patient, while they are still preoccupied with that story, thinking a lot about it, sometimes even losing sleep when internally retelling themselves this emotionally moving episode. The person to whom they may turn should be a colleague who is also a friend, a person they can trust, one who is able to listen with empathy and to react in a supportive way. Sometimes their story can be very personal. It may include an account of professional mistakes, guilt and shame.

"Can two walk together, except they are agreed?" (Amos, 3, 3). The prophet was talking about the Grand Scheme, about the fact that all comes from a divine source. Divine or human, we may view this question as meaning that two people have a common need, and trust each other to fulfill it, walking together down a difficult path supporting each other along the way. Such a mutual relationship creates a comfortable interpersonal space, a space that Winnicott describes as open to play and creativity, where the two can walk together, stimulating personal and professional growth and development.

It also should be pointed out that only a few senior physicians and psycho-therapists still have formal supervision, hence the importance of this book. The book deals with the narratives of two therapists: a clinical psychologist working in psychotherapy, and a family physician (GP), who is a practitioner of bio-psycho-social medicine. Both have had long-term relationships with their patients or clients and with one another. In a day's work, both listen to human suffering, and both work to ease pain and heal. As close friends, they are able to write openly to one another about special cases, especially those with patients who touched them emotionally. Such interpersonal relations were often the source of many reflections, afterthoughts, questions, self-awareness, insights, sometimes involving ethical considerations, conflicts and dilemmas. The writing, and waiting for the reaction of the other, were times of intense feelings, often bringing about further associations, with one story leading not only to an understanding comment, but also to a new, somehow similar, narrative.

The writing of letters is a well-known form of communication, often turning into published literature. It was not long ago that letters were handwritten and mailed, and many such collections have been printed, shedding light on the intimate feelings and experiences of such correspondents as Goethe and Eckermann, Rosenzweig and his lover, or between Freud and Fliess, Jung, and Rolland. Because of their very personal nature, these letters were often published posthumously.

Formulating a letter, writing a story that should be read by another person is often a very helpful process for the writer. When writing a story-as-letter, we usually try to relate experiences, thoughts, emotions, and fears clearly, in a comprehensible manner. Every story has an order of subjects and content, an internal coherence. This does not always follow common logic, and often develops according to a "private, subjective logic."

I should now like to reflect upon the place and value of language. Language may be the foremost line of demarcation between humans and animals. All humans speak a language, yet there is not one language that all humans speak.

However, there is something hidden in language – in every language – something that can neither be said nor uttered verbally so that language only approximates what we want to express. Also the other – listener or reader – has their own personal language. If they are open, tuned in and ready to listen, listeners or readers will be able to understand the language that was used and spoken, to translate it into their own personal language.

In Israel we have an additional problem. We are a pluralistic, multicultural society of immigrants, who grew up with different mother tongues and learned Hebrew (our common language) later in our lives. Patients and therapists are usually more at ease when they come from the same culture and speak the same language, although this is not always possible. Thus, both sides have to learn to understand the other and subjectively translate what they understand.

Furthermore every profession has its culture and terminology (language). Therefore, one has to translate the words that one reads or hears, several times, and on different levels.

Barriers such as cultural background and specific professional terminology may be a reason that letter writing is sometimes easier than direct dialogue. It is often easier to say something emotional, aggressive (perhaps hurtful), intimate or loving when we do not have to face the object of our emotions and are thus oblivious to their mimics and nonverbal expressions. Speaking on the telephone may allow us to be focused on the other's voice only, maybe comfortably preventing us from personally interacting and relating. In a letter one is able to "speak" to the other without interruptions and immediate reactions, one can write a whole exposure of one's personal narrative. One can write in the hope (or illusion) that the other will agree and react positively.

Therapists and physicians may also enter a new and unknown area with their patients, or sometimes discover, by associations and sensitivity, that the relationship with a certain patient had opened up unknown and undiscovered parts in their own psyche. These new discoveries might be astonishing, moving, or even frightening for them. They need an empathic, understanding, supportive person, who can be trusted, with whom they can share their experiences, emotions, and reflections.

As I have mentioned, in some therapeutic professions, formal supervision may be used for these purposes. Other therapists may have an opportunity to talk about the relationship with some significant patients in a Balint group situation. This book presents an interaction between two equals, who alternate the dynamic roles of writer and reader-reactor.

Philosopher Martin Buber drew our attention to the fact that a dialogue reveals things that would have never been discovered in a monologue. Thus, by turning to the other and trying to deliver my message to him or her, I can deepen my knowledge about myself. I am able to know more, not only about the other, but also (and especially) about myself. Emmanuel Levinas added a new dimension to the dialogue by emphasizing one's responsibility for the other. When one has an encounter with "another," and certainly when one starts to communicate with this other person, one becomes morally responsible for that person. When two therapists tell each other stories about treatment, this very dialogue broadens the scope and perspective of the treatment that they have given. The dialogue between two storytellers (therapists) is stimulating, dynamic, moving, enhancing, and creative for both of them. They may realize that their stories are aimed also at "third parties" (other professionals, the public). Thus, a dynamic triangle will develop between the two authors and the reader.

I was the first reader of these treatment narratives and I would like to relate to some issues and point out the impact of these narratives on me. Generally, we deal here with impressive illustrations of the various aspects of the doctor (physician and/or psychologist)–patient relationship. The authors describe episodes that had partly happened in reality (in the "here and now" of the office or at-home visit), during the encounter with a patient and his/her family. Partly they had happened on the level of transference: what this encounter had awoken associatively in their memories and recollections of former life experiences. Such a process can happen either in the psyche of the patient or in that of the therapist (the therapist's counter-transference).

One can also describe these relationships in humanistic, existentialist terms, as we deal here with relationships on two levels – that of patient–therapist (or physician) and that of two therapists engaged in an open and honest dialogue about what had happened in their relationship with a patient. They reflect on a number of "right" and "wrong" decisions that they had made, and they struggle with dilemmas. These are not easy memories and experiences, as it is not easy to take responsibility for what has been said or done. But it is important that while bearing this responsibility, one is not alone, one has the possibility to share these with an empathic and supporting other.

This is not a systematic teaching book of therapeutic skills or methods, but it is a treasury of stories that lead the reader to look into the world of emotions, dilemmas, and open questions in the two clinicians' ongoing relationship with their patients.

Those who would like to learn more of what happens once the door is closed, and therapist and patient meet, will benefit from these fascinating stories and may identify with certain parts of them and perhaps later use them in their own personal or professional life. Finally, reading this book of human interactions is in itself a process of learning through experience, an enrichment of one's own personality.

Professor Benyamin Maoz
January 2007

This book consists of a series of case histories written by two doctors, a general practitioner and a psychotherapist, who are good friends. At the end of each account there is a brief response from the co-author. A third friend, a psychiatrist from a slightly older generation provides a sympathetic but more objective commentary. I can sense the warmth of feeling that these three have for each other.

I am also aware as I read the stories that these are no ordinary case histories. First of all they all describe the patient as a live human being with feelings and relationships. Sometimes they are seem to be looking us in the face and telling their own stories so that we forget that the doctor is even there as an intermediary. But mostly we are very much aware that the doctor's own experience of the relationship is equally important. Stanley and André are doing what William Carlos Williams called 'telling doctor stories'. Williams was both a family physician and a major modern poet. His descriptions of his encounters with his patients reveal some of the powerful feelings they aroused in him and almost certainly helped him to deal with his emotions.

Two other important figures in the charting of the doctor-patient relationship were Michael and Enid Balint who pioneered seminars for general practitioners to help them to understand their patients and themselves. Enid Balint has written that, in order to understand what is going on, the doctor has to be able to identify with the patient – and then withdraw from the identification to become once more an objective professional observer. The second phase is not so easy, especially if doctor and patient have discovered that they have a genuine affinity for each other. This may be based on experiences they have in common; or less obviously it may reflect an emotional resonance. Sometimes you look at another person and see an aspect of yourself gazing back at you. If the patient's behaviour expresses attitudes that the doctor has tried to disown in himself, there will be trouble ahead! As Dr Williams once said to one of his students: 'there's nothing like a difficult patient to show us ourselves'.

The doctor-patient stories in this book give evidence of the doctors' devoted care. And yet we often find them troubled or even distressed. They reflect on some of their clinical judgments and wonder if the decisions have been influenced by the doctor's own emotional needs. Sometimes they feel angry and humiliated as a result of a patient's 'manipulation'. They are touched deeply by accounts of love, loss, loneliness, betrayal or decline. Like many of their patients they have suffered the dislocation of being immigrants. They confess to the sensations aroused by an attractive patient ('The girl from Ipanema', as André puts it to Stanley) and then feel guilt stricken despite their exemplary behaviour. They are confronted with reminders of their own need to be healers: especially when a patient stubbornly refuses to be healed.

Towards the end of each story we find the doctor groping his way towards insight into his own reactions. His friend and colleague then adds a few words of comfort, support, insight and recognition. I have the impression that feeling deeply about at least some of one's patients is not only inevitable and potentially painful but in the interests of good clinical care. We need to know where the boundaries are and to respect them on the whole, but an occasional crossing to the other side can be beneficial. At the end of the book we are treated to some calm wisdom from Dr Ben Maoz, as he reflects on the feelings aroused and reminds us of the ethical issues.

I greatly enjoyed this book and felt at the end that I had learned a good deal, not least about myself. I think it might do the same for you.

John Salinsky
March 2007

References

Williams W Carlos ed. Robert Coles (1987) *The Doctor Stories.* Faber and Faber, London.

Elder A and Samuel O (eds)(1987) *While I'm Here, Doctor: a study of the doctor-patient relationship.* Tavistock Publications, London and New York.

About the authors

Dr Andre Matalon is a family physician with over 25 years of experience. He was born in 1953 in Cairo, Egypt, but from the age of four years he moved to Sao Paulo, Brazil, with his family. In 1975, at the age of 21 years, Dr Matalon immigrated to Israel where he completed, with honors, his medical training at the Tel Aviv University. He teaches at the Sackler's School of Medicine of the Tel Aviv University courses for undergraduate medical students and postgraduate residents in Family Medicine and for the last 10 years has been a lecturer in the Department of Family Medicine of Tel Aviv University where he is responsible for the psychosocial teaching for residents in Family Medicine. Furthermore over the past three years he has held the position of head of the Department of Family Medicine at the Rabin Medical Center in Petach Tikva. In this post he is responsible for the residency program for Family Medicine at the Tel Aviv and Dan-Petach Tikva districts of Clalit Health Services, the biggest health maintenance organization in Israel.

Presently Dr Matalon is practicing Family Medicine in a rural, agricultural village in central Israel. Following his interests, he has also developed an innovative counseling clinic for psychosomatic illnesses. This unique clinic is already well known in Israel and its findings have been presented at different professional conferences all over the world, while scientific papers about the unit have been published in prominent journals of family medicine. To supplement his training, Dr Matalon also completed the School of Psychotherapy of Tel Aviv University.

Dr Matalon is one of the founders of the Israel Balint Society and has lately been elected president of that society which aims at improving the doctor–patient relationship, as well as the integrative and relational aspects of health.

Over the years, Dr Matalon has written over 30 professional publications and took part in writing a book entitled *The Doctor, the Patient and Their Interactions: an introduction to relational medicine* (Maoz B, Rabin S, Katz C, Matalon A. Tel Aviv, Israel: Ramot Publishers, University of Tel Aviv; 2004 [in Hebrew]).

Dr Matalon's professional interests include the relationship of body and mind, stress management, psychosomatics, narrative medicine, mental health in primary care, integrative medicine, meditation and Buddhist philosophy.

Dr Matalon is married, with three children and lives in Petach Tikva, Israel.

Dr Stanley Rabin is a clinical psychologist with over 30 years of experience as a psychotherapist and supervisor in psychotherapy. He was born in South Africa, and received his training and education at the University of Cape Town. In 1975 he immigrated to Israel where he has held many senior posts in a diversity of health and academic facilities including the Mental Health Center in Beersheba; Shalvata Mental Health Center in Hod Hasharon; Israel Defense Forces Medical Corps; Air Force Medical Unit; Occupational Health and Rehabilitation Institute in Raanana; and the Department of Family Medicine, Tel Aviv University.

Presently, Dr Rabin is in private practice in Raanana, Israel. He is a senior lecturer in the Psychiatric Division of the Faculty of Health Sciences, Ben Gurion University of the Negev, Beersheba, Israel. Furthermore, he serves as a senior psychologist in the Department of Psychiatry, Soroka University Medical Center, Beersheba, Israel. His work includes individual psychotherapy, supervision of health professionals, applied research and leader of groups for doctors and health personnel. He is one of the founders of the School of Psychotherapy, Faculty of Health Sciences, School of Continuing Medical Education, Ben Gurion University of the Negev, and is also an active member of the teaching team in the school.

Dr Rabin has written over 60 professional publications over the years and has been involved in writing two books entitled:

- Maoz B, Rabinowitz (Rabin) S, Herz M, Katz C. *Doctors and Their Feelings: a pharmacology of medical caring*. New York: Praeger Press; 1992.

▶ Maoz B, Rabin S, Katz C, Matalon A. *The Doctor, the Patient and Their Interactions: an introduction to relational medicine*. Tel Aviv, Israel: Ramot Publishers, University of Tel Aviv; 2004 (in Hebrew).

Dr Rabin's professional interests include the relationship of body and mind, post-trauma, mental health and primary care, and integrative psychotherapy. He is on the committee of the Israel Balint Society and an Israeli representative to the International Balint Federation. Dr Rabin is married, with three children and lives in Raanana, Israel.

Acknowledgments

We want to express our deep gratitude to Dr John Salinsky, an exceptional London family physician, humanist and writer, for his suggestions, encouragement and help in editing this book. We feel privileged and touched by his friendship.

Special thanks

Our deepest appreciation to our colleague, friend and mentor, Professor Benyamin Maoz, for his valuable contribution and guidance. With his comments and foreword he enriched not only our book, but also our lives.

Permissions

The following publishers gave us permission to publish parts or adaptations of two of our narratives in Chapter 14 and Chapter 15:

1 Georg Thieme Verlag Publishers for "Abuse, freedom, and me," Chapter 14. Article published by Rabin S, Maoz B, Matalon A. Narratives and medicine. *Balint Journal*. 2004; **5**: 18–23.

2 American Psychological Association for "The helper's helplessness: Enrique's story," Chapter 15, adapted from the article "Helpless" published by Matalon A. In *Families, Systems & Health*. 2004; **22** (3): 383–7. Copyright © 2004 by the American Psychological Association. Reprinted (or adapted) with permission.

Dedication

This book is dedicated to our wives Barbara and Estela, that with their encouragement and faithful friendship we could have passed the evenings and nights writing in front of our computers. We had their hearts and minds to reflect on our cases, our dilemmas and our stories, so they are also part of this book. We feel privileged and in deep gratitude for their love and their company in our life journey.

Introduction

Andre Matalon and Stanley Rabin

Two very close friends – a clinical psychologist (SR) and a family physician (AM) – decide to correspond quite spontaneously with one another via email, each from his vantage point in the therapeutic realm. What was our motivation for doing this? Perhaps this indicates, more than anything, our willingness to share, to be listened to and most importantly to reflect. The work of clinicians in most areas of the health field is stressful and overwhelming and often very lonely. These factors and others encouraged us to negotiate some very intimate professional moments with one another, each of us reflecting, from his unique perspective, on the dilemmas, doubts, struggles, and rewards of treating our patients.

Through our correspondence we were able to choose issues/dilemmas which we found interesting. Often it meant that we had to consider, in our practices, which cases or problems were fit to discuss. This injected interest in our work and gave us a different perspective on it, as detachment and looking-on can, in and of themselves, have therapeutic advantages.

Our correspondence is more a correspond-dance than just the exchange of letters. Each essay may have had an impact at the subconscious level of the other and triggered a new response essay. The more we practiced it, the more we became alert and in tune with our feelings and experiences as well as those of our patients, and we two performed a better "tango". These essays exemplify the relational aspects of our clinical work – the interpersonal relationship and its influence on the process of care, and probably on the outcome as well. Growth and development come just slowly, step by step.

The intellectual base of medicine or psychology, the evidence-based protocols and guidelines for physicians, are easily acquired. But for this knowledge to be effective, it must be transformed into common behavior through the emotional knowledge, a subconscious knowledge, and a transformation process that is described in these essays. Intellectual knowledge leads to "doing" while emotional knowledge leads to "being." Both are essentials in caring, and the merging of the two is the real wisdom.

While intellectual knowledge is acquired through learning and memorizing, emotional knowledge is gained through experience, through trial and error, but especially through awareness of our inner soul. Feeling the pain of one's errors and mistakes, feeling one's attractions, compassion/passion about patients, or one's awe and humility at patients' strengths and disappointment in their rejections, are some of the issues touched upon in our correspondence. Experiencing one's helplessness and hopelessness in front of a dying patient who through the years of accompaniment became your friend, one's sadness in the wake of the disability of an old grandfather after suffering a stroke, feeling humble in front of the patient who knows much more than you do about the disease that is taking over his body and soul, are also issues described. Furthermore, our correspondence touches on how the clinician is influenced by external events and its impact on his/her caring.

This emotional knowledge is the difference between being just a good clinician and a true healer. This knowledge is acquired not only by learning but also emotionally; reacting to oneself and acquiring the appropriate personal insight induces in one the universal inherent ability to heal through compassion and hope. All of these questions and dilemmas are related in these essays in a narrative mode. They highlight the process, the feelings that are part of both partners in the clinical encounter, no matter what the cause or the trigger is, or the discomfort that brought them together. Sometimes the focus is on the patient, sometimes on the clinician and sometimes on the environment, as all of them are part of the integrative interactive narrative, influencing the relational aspects of the process.

The cases and the situations here described are real but the identity of the patients and their families was disguised or significantly changed out of respect for their privacy. In saying this, it is clear that it could be impossible for some persons not to identify themselves with some stories or part of them as they are both unique and universal. We are in deep debt and respectful gratitude to all our patients and especially to those whose stories are reported in this book, for the opportunity they gave us to understand human beings but especially to grow and understand ourselves. We think that more than exposing our patients, we are exposing ourselves, in our dilemmas, in our weakness, helplessness and anxieties, but also in our insights, joys and pleasures in doctoring.

We hope that doctors and therapists will enjoy these stories through identification or emotional joining and others will have the opportunity to have a glimpse of the heart and mind of their doctors and therapists.

Our theme is that there is no medicine or psychology on its own – each encounter, each consultation, is a dialogue between two souls, both of them with a past history, with a psychological narrative, with a cultural background, with love, hate, attraction, rejection. We think that we have found the central theme of our correspondence, of our book – relational medicine – relational encounters – relational healing!

CHAPTER 1

Good luck or good judgment?

Andre Matalon

Wolf (Zeev) is an 80-year-old German Jew, very meticulous and preoccupied with his health and appearance. We had endless consultations for his nose which ran "but just after eating," and for the streaks on his nails that he thought were due to a fungus infection. Sometimes, when he was especially anxious, he would not shake hands, worrying about infecting his partner, so responsible and rigidly "correct" he had to be. Although he was a wealthy married man, and father of two married children, without these anxieties he could have been a pleasant and happy person. We often talked about his feelings of loneliness and the euphemistic "golden" days. He came to Israel before World War II, so that he did not live in Germany during the Holocaust. He clearly remembered his parents' depression following their immigration and their disillusionment with the hot, "Levantine" atmosphere of Palestine before the creation of the state of Israel. Both Wolf and his wife made special efforts to maintain their "European way of life" and both took valium for a "good" sleep.

One month before the event I would like to present, Wolf was hospitalized – for the first time in his life – for elective prostate hypertrophy surgery. Following the operation he went into prolonged delirium with several nights of irritability and unrest. The staff of the Urology Ward felt that they had to bind his hands and feet to his bed in order to prevent him from pulling out his catheter and his intravenous line.

When they came to see me after the hospitalization, both Wolf and his wife were shocked and overwhelmed by what had happened to him. He was depressed and did not want to eat or talk and expressed his wish to die. He felt that after going through these experiences life was not worth living. I felt we had a good and supportive talk, and I was about to suggest an antidepressant, as I had previously thought that it could help him and I was waiting for an opportunity. However, when checking his blood pressure I was surprised to find an atrial fibrillation irregular pulse. Suddenly, I was in conflict, facing multiple dilemmas – do I send him back to the hospital or do I treat him? Should I conceal the diagnosis or reveal it? The hospital discharge letter gave no clues as to how long he had had atrial fibrillation, although in retrospect, it could have been the cause of the prolonged delirium. But he felt good, there were no signs of heart failure or distress, and he was unaware of the problem. He was just bothered by his depression and pain when urinating. Sharing my diagnosis with him and his wife, we decided to treat him at home and try to arrange an echocardiograph and a cardiologic consultation. In the meanwhile I put him on anticoagulant therapy (coumadin) as atrial fibrillation can cause blood clotting inside the heart chambers.

Three days later, his first anticoagulation INR-PT test was 2 after 5 mg of coumadin a day, and we were all satisfied with the result (the normal range of INR test in coumadin-treated patients is between 2 and 4). He forgot the depression as he had a new health anxiety to be preoccupied with. On the next blood test, three days later, the laboratory clerk urgently called me, telling me that his INR-PT test was 10! Once again, I faced the same dilemma I had faced only a few days earlier – send him back to hospital or call him immediately and stop his medication. Despite my growing anxieties, I chose the second option, after receiving reassurance that he would immediately go to the hospital if he had either a fall or a bruise, as there was a risk of serious bleeding. I urged him to come to see me in two days to continue our monitoring. In the meantime he had had his echocardiogram and consulted with the cardiologist who was in total agreement with my decision to treat him with coumadin and did not offer any new alternative treatment.

Two days later, I was happily driving to my surgery when my eyes caught a death notice with his Hebrew name on it (Zeev) and the funeral being this very day and hour. I was blinded by my own anxieties and almost choked. I imagined myself coming to the mourners, trying to explain the rationale of the risk I took by not sending him to hospital based on his bad experiences and suffering when tied down to his bed, one month previously. I felt that I had exercised wrong judgment for the sake of his dignity!

From that moment on, I could hardly work. The first thing I did when entering the surgery was to check if he was in my appointment list of scheduled patients, and he wasn't. My thoughts wandered, and I examined my inner feelings to see whether I had had an unconscious desire to get rid of him, and that this desire may have blinded me from seeing the risks. But I couldn't find a justification for these thoughts. I could really feel my compassion for his suffering and my fight for his dignity and well-being. How could I suggest "preventive" hospitalization after the traumatic experience he had? How could I suggest a "preventive" hospitalization when he was totally asymptomatic? I kept asking myself whether I would treat him in the same way again, but I had no answers.

Two hours later, Wolf just came in without an appointment and could not understand my intense burst of sympathy and welcome. He felt perfectly well and we scheduled the next blood tests and coumadin treatment. I didn't tell him about my fears and thoughts over the past few hours. I could not resist asking him if there were other persons in his neighborhood with his name. He answered that his name and family name are almost as widespread as Cohen, and that he is always bothered by telephone calls searching for the other Wolf (Zeev).

I keep asking myself if I would do it again, but I still have no answers. Was it a case of good luck or good judgment?

Dear Andre,

Your case touched me. You took a calculated professional decision which I can well understand and admire. The other point that struck me is the element of surprise – the sudden change in your story. As in a suspense movie, it was as if you were reliving him, bringing him up from the grave. What a twist and how emotive it was.

Have a good week.

Stan

Hi Stan,

Thanks for your comments.

I took risks for the sake of the patient and his care. Do we do it often? – How much do we do it without being aware of the risks involved for the patient and for ourselves? Is it a feeling of omnipotence or is it our caring and compassion for his suffering that impels us to this behavior?

Andre

CHAPTER 2

Changes, moves, adaptations, and me

Stanley Rabin

Chen is a 28-year-old man who came to see me again today because of anxiety and unexpected mood swings. He is not married, is painfully shy and decidedly heterosexual. Chen is a short person, somewhat overweight, with a kind, boyish and round gentle face; he makes excellent contact but clearly exhibits low self-esteem. He was very lucid in his expression and open about himself.

Chen has never had a long-term relationship with a woman, and came to see me today because of this and because of his acute anxiety symptoms. He told me that he came from a relatively stable family. His mother, a woman whom he described as having much potential, had reconciled herself to being a housewife all her life, looking after him and his 34-year-old divorced sister. His father, of Iraqi background, cares for Chen's material needs, but was somewhat emotionally blunted. The father had difficulty expressing feelings having been raised on an Israeli moshav, worked in the agricultural sector for a time, went to university where he received a degree in civil engineering, and worked for a very prominent international building firm. Because of the father's job, the family had lived overseas several times, accounting for Chen's life story changes, his moves, adaptations, and life separations. Chen was born in Israel, moved to Singapore when he was 6, returned to Israel at age 10, and then lived with his family in the USA from the age of 14 to 16. He returned to Israel for his last two years of high school and then made the next move to the army. Chen's adaptations to these stages were very complicated. He often became anxious, his anxiety always expressed in the somatic form of stomach cramps and nausea, which have accompanied him all his life. "I could not stomach all these changes, readjustments, realignments, connecting, and disconnecting," he said to me on one occasion. Therefore these changes, moves, adjustments, and readjustments became a motif that was very much part of his life trajectory. At this stage I wondered about his family picture, and how and why the frequent separations were so much part of this family story. It later turned out, after taking a family history, that transits and realignments were part of this family's multigenerational separations, coping with loss and then making appropriate readjustments. Chen's mother was born in a refugee transit camp in Europe after World War II. Each of her parents had been married and had children before the war, and both had lost their spouses and children who were murdered in the Holocaust.

Chen's mother imbued her children with a feeling of transition, of life not being permanent, a feeling that Chen had felt all his life. This was felt in his childhood years in Israel and Singapore, again during his early adolescence in Israel, and then in the USA and later throughout his army service. He had the feeling of being in a temporary zone, not really belonging; a feeling of being a fly on the wall. "Was I accepted? What are they thinking of me? Am I good enough?" was his constant concern.

He also had to be the "good child," the healthy one, who had to compensate for all his parents' losses and sadness – Chen's mother had miscarried twice before his sister was born. After Chen was born she had a stillborn child, and then she gave birth to an autistic and severely retarded son. Chen remembers his brother exhibiting autistic-like behavior, rocking, and vomiting. He also recalled how his brother often had chronic ear infections and occasional temper tantrums. Other members of his extended family suffered from manic-depression disorder. "My sister and I turned out to be the only children who were normal: it seems as if I have no normal relatives," he once said to me painfully. "This made me feel even more exceptional and self-conscious." There was never a feeling of permanency in his life. He described his family as "nomads on the go," and then revealed that his maternal grandfather was a capo in a Nazi extermination camp.

His mother was brought up on Holocaust stories, and its horror and tragedy were very much part of Chen's upbringing. Added to this was his mother's exceptional sensitivity to changes, her overprotection, her constant concern with health matters and her general, catastrophic worry. Chen felt that his role in the family dynamics was to protect his mother from further tragedies. Chen's father, however, was insensitive to his son's needs, self-involved in building up his career with travel being very much part of his occupational story. Chen was unable to share his difficulties with his father, and – being his mother's protector – he was also unable to expose his feelings and conflicts to her, as he was careful in trying not to overburden her, wanting to be "the perfect son." At the same time he admitted to feeling suffocated by his mother's over-concern.

After his military service in a special combat unit, he moved out and rented a flat with friends in the city, referring to this move and to making the break as the "correct decision." He had cousins in the UK, and decided to leave Israel to find his way to his own personal freedom in London. Chen's move to the UK after the army and his five-year sojourn there were seen by him as a very important move, one in which he finally asserted his own identity, autonomy, independence, and individuation. But it was also seen as the continuation of his constant search for something else, something whole. He craved personal contact, stability, and tranquility, all of which he had never attained in his childhood, and searched for these things in London. However, this was not to be.

It is true that he studied at the university, got a degree in economics and for a while worked in a prominent financial bank. He did meet a few women but these relationships were not longstanding. He told me that he was always overcome with fear of "not doing the right thing." Women made him feel anxious. After a while he felt estranged, empty and relation-less. He started to consume alcohol, and drinking helped him tone down his frequent, unbearable anxiety symptoms. He also ate excessively and compulsively during his residence in the UK. He slowly became more and more isolated. Besides infrequent dates, he closed himself from the world, content to find his personal pleasure in reading, overeating, watching pornographic films, and masturbating. This went on for a long period of time until he decided to return to Israel again. Returning to Israel was also seen as a way of redefining himself and his belongingness and identity, after feeling quite alienated in the latter years of his stay in the UK.

Back in Israel, Chen's first desire was to return to the UK. He perceived Israel negatively. It was obvious that he was soon ready to make another move – he wanted immediate satisfaction and had a very hard time coping with frustration. These feelings were also part of his relationship with women – when women were serious, he edged away from them, but when they were unattainable he was neurotically drawn to them.

Chen has found work in corporate banking and is slowly readapting. I am very fond of him, happy to see him on my list once a week. He seems to have benefited from our relationship, attempting to come to terms with his many conflicts, trying to cope with his present situation and struggling with his past intra-psychic conflicts.

Yet I wonder about this case. As I sit back in my psychotherapist's chair I ponder my helping role very seriously. Will I, as a psychotherapist, fulfill his wishes of having someone at his side, someone who will be supportive and caring? I then ask myself: How do changes in my life affect me personally? I changed apartments six times, moved to three cities in Israel, changed jobs several times. How did these changes impact my family and me? And now, with Israel in crisis in the throes of the second Intifada, people around me are talking of leaving the country, breaking bonds, friendships, lifelong relationships. A sudden feeling of sadness overwhelms me. My mind goes back to further changes I have made myself, in my life as a new immigrant to Israel. I relive my sadness at seeing my elderly father at the Cape Town harbor softly waving me off goodbye, me to my new beginnings as I sailed away to my new country, leaving him and my mother behind, both of them devastated at saying goodbye to me. I suddenly have a picture of him, lonely and sick, probably eaten up with longing and yearning for his only son across the seas, while leaving me to address my own guilt. As I take stock of my past I dare to ask if it was all worth it. Do ideals overcome personal responsibility? Can love for a country or an ideal overshadow the love for a loved one?

Dear Stan,

Your story took me back to my own history. As you know I also left my parents when I was 20 years old for an ideology. Simply stated, I came to Israel under the influence of the Zionist movement. Nowadays I can also understand that, apart from it, there were other reasons. Firstly the need for "freedom," an individuation task of "late adolescence." But I came also in search of roots. As you know I was born in Egypt, we spoke French at home, and we even sang "La Marseillaise." But when I was three years old my family was forced to emigrate to Brazil. And now, there is still in me (and I hope that this will never fade) the longing for a good coffee, the thrill of a good game of football, and the excitement of a beautiful woman (the girl from Ipanema) passing by me.

But I can also see in your story a protective father trying to soothe the moves in the life of your patients. You also had a lot of passages in your life, I had too, and we both did them by ourselves, with little financial support from our parents. But also they made their passages throughout life probably without sufficient guidance from their own parents. I remember you telling me that your father moved from Lithuania to the United States and from there to South Africa. My father also did the same by moving from Turkey to Egypt where he lost his father when he was 12 years old and then to Brazil when he was 40, and finally to Israel after his retirement. By your supporting and treating Chen you are going through your own corrective emotional experience.

Have a nice evening.

Andre

Dear Andre,

Thanks, Andre, for your comments — I now have a few more insights. I agree that my relationship with Chen is very much a father–son relationship. I sometimes felt too much concern for him and was decidedly overprotective of him. I now also realize that not only you, Andre, did I consult with. I also chose to discuss him with another colleague at an informal consultation session recently. Why has Chen such a special significance for me? In many instances in my practice I am a father figure to many of my young male or female patients. They generally have positive feelings towards me too and the relationship is very warm and supportive. But then I ask, maybe I overprotect them or become clingy to them, not wanting to let them go because of my own guilt? After all, I myself was a parental child, probably like you, and learned to be a parent at a very early age, while being an informal caregiver to my very loving, but financially burdened parents throughout their lives. It is no surprise that I, and maybe you too, chose the helping health profession. Even though we financially struggled as a family, my parents did give me emotionally what I needed. I saw my dad a few times after I immigrated (even though he was then sick and blind) which is some consolation to me. My mother, as you remember, immigrated to Israel shortly after my father passed away and lived a very full and happy life until she passed away in 1998. So maybe, in a way, I was giving to Chen a little of the good family life he never had.

As I write these words to you, I now make a further discovery. I realize that with me the changes, moves, separations are not only the physical changes involved in acculturation, or realignment as Chen's case so poignantly illustrated. It is also my own coming to terms with something else, a much deeper part of myself. The sadness involved in coming to terms with my internal changes, the loss of my youth, my parents, my past as I enter a new phase in my personal life cycle.

Warmest regards,

Stan

CHAPTER 3

To treat or not to treat, that is the question!

Andre Matalon

Tzivia is a 67-year-old woman, born in Yemen. She is the mother of five children and she is illiterate. Five years ago, her husband Zechariah had a severe road accident that took away his ability to work, leaving him handicapped and bankrupt. When I first met Zechariah he was confused and disoriented and I could not diagnose either a possible depression or post-traumatic stress disorder. After treatment with various antidepressant medications, and with the passage of time, it became clear that Alzheimer's disease was taking over his brain and soul. Sometimes I thought that this disease could be a blessing – it meant he did not have to feel any pain, despite his difficulties in walking because of his plated femur, and his back, curved with innumerable vertebral fractures. He visited me at the request of his attorney who wanted to "inflate" his medical file. Although Zechariah had sad eyes, he was always glad to see me; he answered my questions with kindness but not always appropriately. Mostly it was Tzivia who answered the questions for him. For her, he "had to be" in constant pain and suffering. But, in fact, she was the one in constant pain and suffering. She attended the clinic frequently. Never would a week go by without her visiting me, never receiving any relief from the different drugs I prescribed to her.

She was always irritated, angry, and she never looked me in the eye. She complained of headaches, chest pain, dizziness, fatigue, and pain in her joints. She wanted more and more new tests to find a disease that could explain her suffering. No drug would soothe her pain, nor my commitment, devotion and compassion. I became more and more frustrated and my good communication skills seemed useless.

After almost three years with this pattern of visits and consultations, Tzivia decided to tell me what was really in her heart, the "secret pain" that bothered her. She now felt that it was the right time to bare her soul to me; from my perspective, I attributed this timing to the possible growing confidence and trust that she felt in our relationship. After a few seconds of hesitation she told me of her husband "demands" that she engage in sexual activities every night and countless times during the day. In her words she was sure that "he was out of his mind." With the development of his disease and the release of his inhibitions he would, without any judgment, run after her, undress her and "do whatever he wanted." If she refused to comply, he would shout at her and would then go outside, half-naked, telling the neighbors that his wife was not a good wife. She felt constant shame and humiliation and she felt that no one could help her. She was entrapped, angry and humiliated, but could not tell this to her children. It turned out that from the very beginning of their marriage, she was always submissive. When she was 11, her father decided that it was time to marry her off to a cousin, 10 years her senior. For the next 56 years while she dutifully served her husband, she also worked hard as a housekeeper for rich neighbors. Having worked hard all her life, she had thought that when arriving at old age she would be able to rest, or at least her body would – a body, she complained, that had never given her any pleasure.

After this confession she had a further request. She asked me to give her husband a pill that would lessen his sexual drive, a pill that she could dissolve in his coffee, without him knowing. I still don't know why I agreed to her request. Maybe because her suffering touched me, maybe my compassion for her situation or possibly because I thought that by doing so, my own feelings of helplessness would end. It may also have been that her confession touched me. She let me enter into her most intimate inner world. This flattered me and I unconsciously may not have wanted to let her down, to be frustrated and leave me empty handed. I now realize that I did not give a thought to Zechariah. I was totally involved in her story, and I thought only of how I could help her. I then prescribed drops of haloperidol, in a low dose of half a milligram, to be given to him once every evening. I thought (and later rationalized) that it would not be harmful for an Alzheimer patient anyway, since I conveniently related to Zechariah's over-sexual drive as part of his losing judgment and losing touch with reality. I gave her the drug and conveniently forgot about the case.

Two weeks later Tzivia came back and I recognized, within myself, the first signs of inner concern. Of course the drug did not help and Tzivia tried to double the dosage, without discussing this with me. She later asked if she could double it again. Suddenly the inner bells of "danger" were ringing loudly. What would happen if Zechariah developed adverse reactions to the drug, some of these being irreversible? What would happen if he became drowsy from the drug, fell and fractured a bone? How would I explain this to his children? Would they accept my explanation that it was for the sake of their mother? Suddenly, the medico-legal aspects of this case frightened me, and were even greater than my desire to help them with their problems. How could I treat Zechariah without his knowledge and consent? In retrospect, maybe I should have tried to find a custodian for him. It is possible that the issue that bothers Tzivia does not bother him at all. It is probably the only pleasure or pleasant experience left for him to feel. As clinicians, can we decide not to treat this case? Are we allowed to treat one spouse at the expense of the other? To treat him or not to treat him, I kept asking myself.

Now, rethinking the case in a contextual way, I could find good reasons for me to treat him, even if it had to be through his wife. Strengthening her caregiver role could have been a very important issue in his health and not only in hers. She is the only basic informal caregiver who is still feeding him, dressing him, bathing him and will continue to do so until his death, since it is not acceptable in Yemenite culture to place the elderly into an institution of any form. Ethically, I also think it was very reasonable to protect Tzivia from what seemed to be recurrent rape. This systemic thinking, taking into account both the partners, is the best message that can be learned in family practice and helps me a great deal to reframe this case in contextual terms. I became aware that I had to strengthen her role and avoid as much as possible the caregiver burden which has been mentioned recently in the psychological literature.

In this case, I now realize that I may have become overwhelmed by my own inner anxieties and conflicts. I let Tzivia become frustrated, and I became frustrated as well. It was also almost impossible to discuss his sexual appetites with Zechariah in person as he was too far gone. She was not able to discuss any of her problems with her children, and she did not allow me to discuss these issues with any of them, so preventing a shared family decision. She was overwhelmed by her embarrassment and shame. Quite possibly, it was also just a continuation of her submission, of her always being a victim.

And what about myself? What happened to me in the process? Can I live with the knowledge that Tzivia will adjust the dosage of haloperidol according to her needs? Who is the identified patient in this case, Tzivia or Zechariah? And yet, I am still troubled by my previous dilemma: to treat him or not to treat him?

Dear Andre,

Wow, Andre, what a dilemma, and how so beautifully described. I can certainly understand you. It is almost as if you allowed yourself to decide how much sex Tzivia should have, in what dosage and when. I guess we all try to "play God" in our professions at times. I often wonder whether it is not my frustration at not being a film director that allows me to want to direct others' lives. But what alternative did you really have in your case? In your place, I would have done the same thing, and still be left with feelings of frustration and guilt. I also have this kind of dilemma very often in my clinic. I ask myself is it fair that the index patient that comes for treatment is the real patient who should be treated? I often feel frustrated that the real patient will never be seen by me.

I also often look for the "perfect justice" and the "perfect cure," but realize that there is no such thing.

Andre, I felt extremely sad by this case too – for both her and for him. This is the case where culture, family, and illness came together to make us feel humble in front of our professional helplessness in our need to "cure" everything. So, Andre, try and see your case in this perspective.

Your pal,

Stan

CHAPTER 4

Thrills and secrets

Stanley Rabin

Amit is a single man who told me, on his initial visit, that he came to see me because of his fears that "I am like my mother." His mother left him when he was a few months old and went off with her lover, but over the years Amit had seen her occasionally. Amit lived with his father who married a widow with three children. His stepmother treated him very badly. She abused him emotionally and often physically. Amit spent most of his adolescent years with his friends' families. He slept in their homes and was almost "adopted" by many of them. He yearned for affection. Amit was a hyperactive and attractive 28-year-old man. When I first met him, he had just decided to study physiotherapy. He had a girlfriend whom he loved. She adored him and the couple planned to get married. In taking his history I learned of his sensation-seeking behavior. He vividly described how he loved to keep the adrenalin going in his work as an ambulance driver.

MONOLOGUE
I love to do special things, to go on special missions. It gives me a wonderful tingly sensation. The sound of the siren intoxicates me. The lights of the ambulance thrill me. Heavy rock music on the trip to the injured person, plus fast driving, keeps me going more and more. I long for a dangerous mission! They uplift me. Without this kick I feel bored. Then I look for

things to do to keep me searching for new exciting things. Adrenalin is my very being. Watching TV is boring. Visiting Europe is boring for me. I need action.

He later added that the reason for coming for treatment was that he realized how dysfunctional his risk-taking behavior was. This was clearly evident to him when four months previously he traveled to Brazil with a friend. A few days after getting there he hired a 4 × 4 pick-up (he had never driven a jeep in his life) and drove at top speed, like an ambulance driver, until he had an accident. He was slightly injured but was in shock. At that moment he realized that he needed psychological help. As I considered the case I remembered how Amit found the sensation-seeking behavior to be almost sexual (orgasmic). Suddenly this made me reflect about cases I had treated, many men and woman who got their thrills from surprise and sensation seeking. That this behavior has no cultural or religious bounds was well illustrated in the case I remember, treating, many years ago, a 48-year-old ultra-orthodox religious man who had been having a two-decade affair with his neighbor's wife – also religious. The synagogue was their place of rendezvous, their secret meeting place, for arranging and timing their next romantic visit. It was as if they were almost taking risks in the presence of God! Yet my recent case is the one I want to tell you more about.

Andrea, a 40-year-old professional TV reporter, has been in my treatment for almost one year. Recently I have been seeing her with her husband Yaron, a physician in the local hospital. The couple, parents of a 15-year-old son, has had a very stormy and complicated relationship where the wife has often been betraying her husband in a particular way. She was not depressed but suffered from dysphoria and anxiety, especially when her 45-year-old husband Yaron found out about her eight-month special relationship with a rich lawyer she met.

Andrea also suffers, like Amit, from risk-taking behavior. There were many interesting occasions when she, like a film producer, directed her own risk-taking narrative. She would set up thrilling, surprising encounters with her lover at often not so secret places. Fantasies were her game and she did this in a big way! On another occasion, while on a reporting assignment in an African country, she invited her lover to meet her for a secret rendezvous. She got pleasure out of telling him that they were like two secret service agents on a secret mission. Andrea would get particular pleasure out of arranging multiple meetings in various countries in a very short space of time, trying to fit in as much tension into her overbooked schedule, so as to accommodate her lover in her sexual and erotic pleasures! Andrea worked in danger zones, the trouble spots of the world. This gave vent to even more daring escapades! In one event she was reporting in an enemy country for a foreign TV network. She went there incognito and found it quite thrilling to walk among the citizens of this hostile, anti-Jewish country, softly humming Jewish melodies to herself!

One day Andrea came to see me again, this time for a much more serious reason. A week previously she was diagnosed with cancer. The prognosis was not encouraging, and this was well known to Andrea and her husband. She spoke sadly but very rationally to me about the future, well aware of her medical condition. Yaron supported her. As a doctor, he felt comfortable in the role of caregiver, accompanying Andrea on her "medical highway" of tests, visits to specialists, and alternative treatments and involving himself in the chemotherapy treatments which she had at first.

My involvement with the couple was complicated. While I was being put off by the way Andrea had emotionally hurt her husband, I could not but admire her for her compelling brave outlook towards her illness and for her commendable coping skills. Yaron and Andrea had not spoken to their only son about the seriousness of Andrea's illness, something that I counseled them about in a few joint sessions. Notwithstanding Andrea's infidelity, the couple had decided to try to repair their relationship and build up trust once again, and I decided to treat them as a couple. Therapy turned out to be a slow and complicated process. I found myself with mixed feelings. I liked Andrea, her seductive feminine demeanor, her narcissistic smile and her even-tempered presentation of herself and her coping skills. On the other hand I felt uncomfortable in the situation. Yaron had to learn to forgive Andrea for her betrayal, which was not easy for him to do. I identified with Yaron in his physician role, wanting to give, to care for and nurse a sick wife. Yet it was clear to me that he still had ambivalent feelings about their marriage. For me, Yaron was a tragic figure caught up in a delicate life drama. Many thoughts ran through my mind. Could it only be that the illness had brought the couple together, to start licking their marital wounds? Can old wounds be repaired through illness? Was Andrea being punished for her unfaithfulness? Did Yaron unconsciously want to keep Andrea sick and dependent on him – to keep her in the sick role – so as to keep their marriage together?

As they left my office, yesterday, I thought of Andrea. I suddenly felt that, for me, she had lost her sensuality, her vitality, and the sparkle in her eyes. I struggled with my change of feelings, and asked myself whether this change in me was because of her disease or because she had ceased to provide me with the thrill, adventure and excitement that made my practice less ordinary. Do I feel guilty (or even maybe deserve to be punished) for my forbidden thoughts? Do we clinicians live for those excitements, thrills, secrets and romances to fulfill our own needs? Was Andrea so different from many of us, I asked myself? For her, as with Amit, life may only be worth living when there are thrills, excitement, adventures, surprises, love and secrets.

Dear Andre,

After sending you my case I made a further revelation, which I want to share with you. We often need excitement in our professional lives and seek it out. I must admit to you that there is an inner thrill in me sometimes treating very important people, injecting psychological interest and meaning into my often monotonous and lonely professional life. As if I am somehow affecting their achievements, I am part of their lives and successes. I know it is silly but I must admit this to you. So taking risks and keeping patients' secrets in us, in our personal safe and caring hearts, can be very complicated. Don't you think? I would be very interested to hear your response, sometime, when you have time.

Enjoy the weekend,

Stan

Dear Stan,

There is a fine line that separates the emotion of interest, from interest in the emotion. Sometimes this interest is sexually charged, and we cannot deny its existence. We also tend to feel guilty when we realize that our interest can be sexually tinged. We must not allow our guilt to paralyze our thinking, but we must guard against expressing our emotions in ways that may be perceived as exploitative. Your story reminded me of the next story-case, maybe with a similar thrill and excitement, which I want to share with you. Continuity of care in family practice, as in psychotherapy, demands the skills of dealing with patients' dependence. We have not been taught these skills in medical school, as you are taught and analyzed in psychotherapy, so we are always at risk of over-identifying with our patients and colluding with them. Being aware of the counter-transference, and the thrills and emotions that the patient's story is eliciting in you, is not only the first step against being exploitative, but is also the cornerstone of professional caring and compassionate healing.

Andre

CHAPTER 5

Medical voyeurism

Andre Matalon

After Passover I had an avalanche of people in my clinic. It is as if they held themselves healthy during the holidays and then they needed me again to give them a health booster. I sometimes think that I, myself, am the cause of this excessive load of patients. It may be my need to be needed which probably creates or encourages this dependency. For a long time I have had the feeling that I work harder than my colleagues. I then calm myself down by saying that I offer more comfort, more understanding, to the people I serve, which explains why they search me out more than the others. This, I guess, is a thing to be proud of, and not to be blamed for. But when I am overworked I curse myself and come down excessively hard on myself! Yesterday I had an insight that there is another aspect of one's personality that may encourage visits: voyeurism. Being in such intimacy with the persons one treats, one has the opportunity to witness a whole spectrum of family dramas: marital disharmony, unemployment, disease, disability, and personal defeats or successes. Sometimes I feel that I do not need to watch soap operas on TV, since the dramas unfold right in front of me in nearly every patient that comes to see me, even for the more trivial complaints such as backache or urinary tract infection.

One of these patients who came yesterday with a sore throat was Karin, a woman who has been under my care for 20 years. She is now about 45 years old. She lives with her father and works in a bakery. She is not very clever, nor is she so beautiful. Karin has always been very shy, she is not married nor did she go out with men until the last three years when she told me that she was having an affair with one of her married colleagues at the bakery. Then she came to ask me if she could get pregnant from anal sex! "Would you believe this!" I exclaimed to myself. The man she was dating refused to use condoms, and she was afraid of pregnancy so he induced her into having just anal sex. After she told me about her most intimate sexual moments I provided her with basic sexual education – at the age of 45 years! Yet, since she had spoken to me about these issues, I feel that I was "waiting" for her questions, when she sometimes shared with me her fears and escapades. She is afraid and too shy to go to gynecologists, and is almost always fear-obsessed by these issues. After the initial anxieties that followed the first months of Karin's relationship with her lover, life went on for Karin, without more excitement. I was glad for her. It was her first close intimate contact outside her family and I could almost "see" her growing up and developing. She is now paying much more attention to herself and her clothing. She is more assertive towards her employer and is still in her relationship with her friend/colleague. She also looks healthier and visits the clinic less and less.

But, yesterday I had a new insight. Am I having just an interesting voyeuristic attitude towards her and listening attentively to her intimate adventures, or am I giving her the appropriate bio-psycho-social treatment that we so much praise in family medicine? Taking this further I asked myself whether these feelings are to some extent part of everyday doctor–patient encounters. Was there something in me that facilitated her to open to me? Was I the right person, at the right moment for her to ask those questions? Was it my empathy and nonjudgmental attitude that enabled her to go through growth and development? Or perhaps it was a touch of voyeurism in me?

In a flash of insight I said to myself: "She was, certainly, the right person, at the right moment for me to learn!"

Dear Andre,

I have few comments to add. First of all I would like you to be less critical about yourself. We often, as clinicians, tread the thin red line between our own excitement on sharing our patient's story and our own professional duty. I can understand why you called this moving story "professional voyeurism," although there is no voyeurism in this case. Often in our work a sexual issue is presented to us, as they are frequently conflict driven, because it involves lust and basic human drives. Sometimes, it intertwines into our own lives and sexuality but still without threatening our professional competency. This may be one of the things you learned. The awareness and reflective contemplation on these issues are the tuning of your emotional "immune" system to permit the optimal distance with each patient without endangering professionalism.

I also would like to tell you that I admire your openness.

All the best,

Stan

CHAPTER 6

Ethical dilemmas of a psychotherapist

Stanley Rabin

Benjie, a 30-year-old married man, father of two infant twins, lives on a kibbutz. He was referred to me for depression and anxiety, which clearly affected his occupational and family life. He also complained of sudden outbursts of anger towards his 29-year-old wife, whom he loved, a teacher at a regional school. Benjie presented as a handsome, well-groomed man who was guarded in his words, somewhat suspicious at first in his relationship towards me. He was quite demanding, sometimes challenging me, almost fearful that I may not have understood him during every minute of our engagement. Anxieties mixed with sadness were the predominant features seen at first. I sometimes began to feel quite frustrated by him. I felt that he needed constantly to be on guard, to monitor and control his environment, and me.

I am usually quite an empathic person but there was something in his neediness and demanding attitude towards me that bothered me, eliciting in me negative feelings. I decided to overcome these unconstructive feelings by returning to my role as a professional, and I took a very precise history. Taking a history often has helped me dull my feelings, both positive and negative, as I write down my thoughts and order them. This has allowed me to return to my role as a professional, instead of becoming swept away by my emotions. Somehow I felt that his depressive symptoms, explosive outbursts, and bouts of anxiety were atypical to the normal course of his disorder. After going into great detail about the start and duration of his symptoms, it appeared to me that there might be some link between his army service and the start of these extreme emotions. It took me a few sessions to discover that my hypothesis was correct. In the army, Benjie had been a member of a special combat unit.

It was only after the fourth session that he began somewhat hesitantly to talk about his feelings of guilt and remorse during his military service. Hints were thrown about his experiences then, although he was never able clearly to describe these incidents. Yet, even without going into specific details, I found that I was slowly beginning to understand what he was talking about. I gained a clearer perspective in my mind about what he had been through and the traumas he had encountered, especially the tragic killing of a fellow soldier from enemy fire, whose death he witnessed. Looking at the whole picture I made a diagnosis of post-traumatic stress disorder.

Through our relationship and through my deciphering the partial disclosure of the traumatic events, incidents and experiences he encountered, I was able to change my attitude towards him from cautious distance, to empathy. I saw him as he had been 10 years earlier – a 19-year-old young man, with good intentions, a highly motivated soldier who volunteered himself to the unit where he functioned very well. However, when his compulsory service was over, and following his discharge from the military, he became restless, anxious and then depressed. He expressed enormous guilt about things that had taken place at that time. I realized that part of my job was to help him come to terms emotionally with his deep guilt feelings and to reframe the narrative. I tried to "repair" his story by pointing out to him the reasons for him carrying out orders at the time. I pointed out that he could get some solace from the fact that he had performed his duties well. Yet, as I said these words, I felt a pang of remorse. Was I not justifying killing? And what rights have I, as a therapist, to do so? I was even more confused when I discovered that my subtle legitimization had its positive effects. At times, Benjie would relate small details of what he had done and I became quite overwhelmed by his story. Through his catharsis and my subtle way of making his deeds comprehensible to him (and me), his emotional state slowly improved too. His occupational functioning, as manager of the avocado plantation on the kibbutz, improved dramatically, as did his relationship with his supportive and loving young wife and the twins. He found in me a trusting ally. He was genuinely satisfied with the treatment, and in many ways I felt happy that a good therapeutic job had been done. However, I was troubled by the questions – does my therapeutic strategy in this case, where I tried at times to justify his acts, reflect that in psychotherapy, like in the military, the ends sometimes justify the means? What about my own ambivalent feelings about what he had done?

Hi Stan,

I can feel how difficult this case was for you. How this violence permeates every part of our living in Israel! Even doing it in the name of the state, and I am sure that Benjie did it with good will to protect all of us, violence is always not only against the opponent, but also has boomerang effects – it ends up "infecting" you.

Your ethical point is similar to ours, as family physicians, when we simultaneously treat a battered woman and the perpetrator. One day you can help the healing of a "black eye" of the woman and the next day you have to care for the violent husband who is unemployed, depressed, and anxious. How can you be empathic to his story? As with your Benjie, it is very difficult not to take sides, because you also have your own values.

Bye for now.

Yours,

Andre

CHAPTER 7

Memorial Day in the therapist's room

Stanley Rabin

As you know, Andre, here in Israel, we are confronted – unfortunately almost daily – with unexpected surprising and sometimes tragic events. As clinicians, we may directly or indirectly be involved in these incidents and influenced by them in our daily practice, affecting our treatment mode or relationship with our patients.

Today is Memorial Day for the soldiers fallen in Israel's wars. My morning starts with a 50-year-old patient who is in the process of leaving his wife. He talks to me again about the plans he has made, the way he will break the bad news to his wife and his kids, and how he will then go to live with his 38-year-old girlfriend. All this is expressed matter-of-factly, with feelings mainly related to himself and his own narcissistic needs. I feel frozen listening to his intricate future plan and I cannot get over how today, of all days, I have to listen so attentively to someone so involved in himself. I had never thought of him in these terms before but today I do. I try to stay focused as I recount the day we are remembering.

Next was my 46-year-old OCD (obsessive compulsive disorder) patient, suffering from mood swings. The patient walks in telling me again about how his ex-wife has yet again pitted his two children against him. He had just came from school, where he went to give his 10-year-old son a birthday present; he was furious when his son refused to receive his offer, having been told by his mother "to have nothing to do with your father." I think of the day we are commemorating and suddenly, in an unconscious slip, I find myself offering my patient some immediate, practical advice. Actually I just wanted to say: "Enough! Just remember who we are remembering . . . today. OK?"

I recover from my sublimated explosion of anger when I gently usher Carla into my office. Carla is a delightful, attractive 36-year-old mother of three who has been in therapy with me for years. I have in fact acted as a father figure for her, and she really worships me. Two months ago she gave birth to her third son and proudly shows me cute photographs of him. She tells me of her issues/conflicts related to breastfeeding, adaptation to motherhood, and her low post-natal libido, which is affecting her relationship with her husband. On the one hand, I can feel the warmth and calm within myself, comforted with her presence, talking about life, nurturing, feeding, and birth on this day. Yet discussing her lack of sexual drive on this day seems quite inappropriate and makes me feel quite uncomfortable. On the other hand, she is attractive and vivacious. Fantasies on Memorial Day? "Repress! Stop thinking these thoughts! Stop! This is Memorial Day, remember? Remember!"

Next on my list is a 45-year-old businessman who I have been seeing recently for stress management. He has arrived, tape recorder in hand, to do relaxation exercises as one of his ways of reducing his work stress. He briefly reports back to me about the efforts he has made towards changing his irrational thinking, in order to find better ways for decreasing his anxiety. In the quiet of the morning I talk to him (and to the recorder) about regular and steady breathing, "to help you stay relaxed." All the while I am inwardly contemplating the significance of this day, and the insignificance of the work I am now doing!

My 55-year-old female client saves the day. As she sits in "the hot psychotherapeutic chair" I notice that her face is drawn, she is silent and sad. "What happened?" I ask her gently. She then slowly reveals to me how her best friend of over 35 years died a few days ago, and talks about the reactivation of previous losses and deaths, and her great concern for her son in a combat unit. She stresses the great importance of being able to discuss these matters with me. I am the only person with whom she can genuinely discuss feelings, especially since her husband's death in a car accident three years back. She is isolated, sad, weepy, and lonely. "Yes," I say to myself, "this is really the appropriate case for this day." This thought is poignantly exemplified by the two-minute Memorial Day siren, which opportunely goes off while we are in mid-sentence. Both of us quickly jump up and solemnly stand at attention. We both are, of course, well versed in standing at attention and in silence on this day. As I remain upright focusing on the picture on the wall in front of me, I feel relieved. "She will no doubt shed a tear and I will probably join her," I say to myself. "Thank you. You have made my Memorial Day worthwhile!"

Hi Stan,

Nice – so very nice indeed!

It made me reflect on my values for this Memorial Day . . .

I couldn't imagine such an impact on the everyday life of a therapist –

Thanks for this creative dialogue between us . . . a chain of thoughts and remembrance! I will add a story of witnessing and remembrance that I have been struggling with for the last three months, as it was extremely difficult to put it down on paper. I still don't know why, and I am waiting for your contribution.

Love,

Andre

Dear Andre,

Thanks for your prompt response. I am very much looking forward to reading your vignette. About mine, the truth is that it has not been too easy for me to write it either. I feel troubled about touching on such a sensitive, prohibited, almost "sacred" issue like Remembrance Day. I was surprised at myself for even writing it down the way I did. I wonder how other professionals in other cultures relate to these issues. I think that taboo subjects should be also addressed, however uncomfortable it makes us feel. What do you think? In this frame I am very much looking forward to hearing about your new case.

All the best,

Stan

CHAPTER 8

Witnessing trauma remembrances

Andre Matalon

Suddenly, I was caught unprepared. This 78-year-old man, Leo, was asking me to listen to his stories from the Holocaust – "and this one I haven't yet told anyone." It was a special busy day before Passover, and I asked him to come one week later, at the end of the day so I would be able to give him my full attention. I had prescribed Seroxat for him one month previously as I had been doing for the last 10 years around this time of year. Every year, the approaching Holocaust Memorial Day put him in a bad mood and upset and irritated him; two months later he would return to his natural way of being and stop the medication by himself. But this year it was different. He didn't keep his eyes on me, always looking down. Something was wrong, so I had proposed to him that I would be his listener. One week has passed and here he was.

He was very shy, didn't know where to begin, what to say. He may have also been checking me out, testing whether I would be able to listen to his still-to-be-told story. He told me of the Talmud Torah (Jewish religious education) school in Czechoslovakia where he was born and of his father being a Chassid (a religious Jew of the messianic movement) and how, after some years but still before the war, the school was dismantled and the Jews were distributed in regular public schools. Since that time he and some other Jews were to be bullied every day by the stronger and older boys of the school. But he had a gentile Hungarian "goy" friend, Miklosh, who protected him from the bullying. In return, Leo gave Miklosh half of the bread and jam he brought for lunch. Leo's mother was always very suspicious, wondering how he could eat such a big sandwich and still be so thin and underweight.

However, some years later it was this sandwich that saved his brother's life. After the transports began, Leo and his two brothers were taken from their hometown and transferred to a weapons factory in Germany. On arrival they were divided in different rows: the youngest, and Leo among them, were to stay and work at the factory, but his older brother was to be transferred. Everybody said that they were to be killed. Suddenly, Leo noticed that one of the German soldiers was Miklosh. He went to talk to him but Miklosh didn't want to recognize him. But he talked anyway, talked and shouted, and Miklosh didn't answer, but hit him to the floor with his weapon. The next day his brother suddenly reappeared to work in the factory. This was the last time he saw Miklosh.

Two years later they were put on the train to be transferred to Auschwitz. They were loaded onto the cattle cars, without any food or water, and the doors were closed behind them. The train took almost five days to reach Auschwitz and the weaker people perished on the train, dead of thirst and dehydration. Despite their thirst, however, the passengers had been warned by other young people who had already been to Auschwitz not to drink the water from the barrels at the entrance to the camp, as the water was contaminated.

When Leo arrived in Auschwitz he managed to contain his thirst and go directly to his assigned shack after the registration number had been tattooed on his arm. His oldest brother could not resist his thirst and drank from the barrels. That night he woke up with abdominal pain and diarrhea and had to go to the toilets outside the dorms. He went once, twice, and after the third time he didn't come back. Leo was very worried about him. He went out to search for his brother and found him on the cold, snow-covered December ground, on his way back, with no strength left in him to walk the last 10 meters to the huts. Leo tried to help him but had no strength either. He went back in to call his other brother to help him, but when the brothers got outside again it was to see the body of their older brother being dragged away by the neck with a belt to the huge mountain of dead bodies awaiting mass burial.

At this moment his eyes were full of tears and he couldn't stop sobbing. I was also caught with wet eyes, just being there for him, but unable to make any further step, unable to think what's better for him. He continued his saga, telling me how his other brother died very shortly before the Russians reached Auschwitz, and the camp had to be evacuated. All the prisoners were to be transferred to Bergen Belsen by foot, walking, but by then almost all had swollen feet, and no appropriate shoes to wear against the snow and cold; most of them were weak and completely unable to walk. Those who were able to walk were put to walk, and the ones who couldn't continue the journey, or fell down to the earth while walking, were shot dead, not to delay and detain the evacuation. So this way his brother died, by his side, when Leo could no longer help him walk, and he fell to the earth, forever. Leo cannot understand how he continued the march. He cannot understand how he survived this march. He was almost at the edge of his consciousness, coughing blood, 23 kilograms of skin and bones, as he recalls himself when he entered the tuberculosis sanatorium after being rescued by the Americans.

Now, he couldn't stop the flow of his remembrances, but I couldn't listen any more. At the first opportunity I stood up and helped him through the door, to stay there after his departure, crying myself, finding it almost impossible to put all those thoughts and emotions together. Why was he so eager to tell me? Why now? Why this story? I had a vague remembrance of another opportunity when he also asked me to listen one of his stories, about 10 years earlier. He then had told me of the little tricks he had played to survive Auschwitz, the extra bread from the dead, the extra soup broth from a job done for a companion. But now it was different, not a story of survival, but a story of loss, the death of his two brothers, the only family members that he thought would have survived the Holocaust with him, up until the very last days.

I suddenly had an insight that he was maybe preparing his own departure, his own death. He had been visiting me more and more in the last months, he had difficulties with his increasing shortness of breathing because of heart failure. He had diabetes, a new diabetic renal failure and diabetic neuropathic pain in his feet, reminiscent of the pain of frostbite on his feet on the march from Auschwitz and Bergen Belsen. He couldn't stop thinking about it these days, the days preceding Holocaust Memorial Day.

Next day I thought that I was chosen by him to document his stories, but I couldn't write anything beyond the two first lines of this paper. Every time that I began to write, I had an instant burst of tears that I couldn't hold back. Was it a reaction to my own father's new diseases that were made clear to me in the last months? Was it his untold stories? His fears, his anxieties of getting old? Or maybe my own unresolved silly conflict with my brother that distanced him from me and listening to Leo's story had put ours in perspective. I surely was much involved and overwhelmed, but I didn't want to show my tears. I was afraid that he would feel that he had caused me actual suffering. I thought that I had failed to be "the listener" that I offered to be and had broken the narcissistic figure of myself as being a good listener.

But, still thinking whether it was good for him to tell his story, I realize that he had chosen me for that, and it was not a question for him. Although he had always praised the strength of denial and of repressing these thoughts away from consciousness, as a way of healthy coping for him, he was now actively asking me to listen to him.

I was the one who had an open wound in myself, and had to search why I was so sensitive to his story; why it took me two months to be able to write it down.

For me, Holocaust stories of suffering and losses always bring to mind questions about the meaning of life, the significance of our own existence. Although incomparable, and I say this with difficulty, Holocaust stories had always brought to the surface questions and remembrances of my own losses, traumas and pain throughout life.

Hi Andre,

I think that you are witnessing a special moment that every psychotherapist touches on. Does one encourage expression of feelings that have been repressed for so long, repressed for healthy coping in severely traumatized patients, or does this damage the patient? I sometimes feel that we may have vicarious pleasure out of listening to the traumas of our patients and thereby encourage them to speak about them. I often feel the need to delicately balance between our own needs and the needs of our patients, to protect them, and us.

But, reading the story again, I felt as if it was almost you who was living in the camps, as if you yourself were a prisoner in the camps, a prisoner of your own suffering. You became Leo as you told it, taking over his rhythms.

I hope that maybe by your telling me the story you will soothe your own suffering and pain, as Leo told his story to you.

Have a good day,

Stan

CHAPTER 9

Sa'adia and his limping health

Andre Matalon

Sa'adia is a 60-year-old Yemenite Jew who lives in a rural settlement in central Israel. He is married and the father of five children. He has not worked since his forced retirement four years previously, when his body was ripped by a stroke. Since then he comes to my clinic, situated 400 meters up-hill from his house, regularly. He enters limping and breathing heavily. He comes only once a month for his chronic drug prescriptions, but I feel that I have a secret pleasure in seeing him: he is a happy person! He also puzzles me. He is always smiling, good looking, well dressed and always ready for a chat. When the waiting room is full of patients, some quarreling and competing for five minutes of my attention, he is the one always ready to give up his appointment for a crying child or for the sad suffering face of old grandmother Zohara. He talks to everyone in the waiting room, with his heavy, sometimes unintelligible, speech.

But still, something puzzles me. Is he happy because he is drunk, as I noticed on occasion the smell of beer on his breath? Is his happiness real or a cover-up for his stressful life, for his handicap or for his family situation? In my desire to be authentic in my relationships with my patients, I asked him how come he is so happy. He then disclosed that he had had a very difficult life up until his stroke.

He was born in Yemen, the tenth child of 12 brothers and sisters. When he was four years old his mother died of a puerperal infection after giving birth to her last child. When he was seven years old his father died of influenza, an outbreak that sent a great number of people to their deaths in those days in Yemen. This happened just a few days before the family was to immigrate to Israel. Fortunately, his brothers and sisters came to Israel together and they settled in the same rural village. But they were a strange lot. They were certainly not like most Yemenites I have treated; Sa'adia was illiterate. The men in his family were warriors from a mountainous region of Yemen, and not liked by the other Yemenite Jews. They encountered difficulties in adapting to modern Israeli society and failed in many ways. He did not attend school in Israel; and he says that and his truancy were not even noticed by the authorities. He eventually married his cousin Ghahari when she was 16 years old and the first two of their children died of genetic diseases. From the age of 12 he had worked in agriculture, 12-hour workdays that began at 5 a.m. every morning. His wages were scarcely sufficient to provide milk for his children. His wife also had to work as a housekeeper in a nearby city to supplement the family income.

As his children grew, he had difficulty teaching them boundaries, respect and good manners. Two of his children were imprisoned for robbery and drug peddling. He began to drink and smoke heavily to escape his misery. Nothing interested him. Insidious hypertension and diabetes were already seeding their disaster in his body. He chose not to look after himself; he had no money for expensive anticholesterol, diabetes and hypertension drugs and had no drive for life. "I do not feel bad, so why take drugs?" he asked with a defiant smile on his toothless mouth. I was the new doctor, when I first met him, still not trusted by him. In a last effort to help him, the local rabbi offered him a job as a shochet (kosher slaughterer) and after one month of apprenticeship he was ready to work. It paid a small salary, and he still had economic difficulties but the work commanded respect, and was consistent with his warrior and hunter past. But now, even under religious supervision, he was exploited. He worked for long hours for a very low salary, and the rabbis explained that he was doing a mitzvah (commandment or good deed). But hypertension, diabetes, drinking, and smoking had already done their work and Sa'adia did not enjoy even one year of his new job. He fell down one day in a convulsive attack that turned out to be the presentation of a devastating stroke at the age of 56 years. He was hospitalized and in a coma for three weeks, and his partial recovery occurred over a period of one year. His right limbs are still spastic and he has a great difficulty in walking. His speech is also sometimes difficult to understand because of his paralyzed tongue.

But something else happened over these next four years of my follow-up. He began receiving a monthly disability pension from the social services, which was higher than his previous salary. He was then able to fix his teeth and one day he entered the clinic just to show me his new shining smile. He began to learn to read at the local collel (religious school for married men), and turned out to be a good student. He was the youngest of the group and a good singer and rapidly became a valued companion for the older participants. At home things calmed down. Although his two boys still had their problems with the police, all his children left home, married and returned weekly for the Sabbath reunion at his house. Ghahari proudly prepared hamin, jahnun, and kubana and all other traditional Yemenite foods that the grandchildren love. A new, healthier adaptation occurred. Sa'adia now accepted his medications and adhered to therapy; his diabetes and hypertension were well controlled. He found meaning in taking his medicines. "This new life is worthwhile living," he declared. In his deterministic, spiritual way, he accepts his condition. He explains that it is God's wish. God brought to him suffering and redemption through his stroke.

I marvel how healthy this acceptance is: acceptance of suffering and disease as facts of life, as part of existence. This also makes me wonder about my job; sometimes fighting against disease, sometimes relieving suffering and sometimes being a mindful and caring observer of people adapting to their lives.

By working and treating this special rural population over the last five years, I have learned what acceptance is. I have learned to accept the mentally retarded that wander through the village, bringing laughter to some children and fear to others. I have learned to accept the smile of the simple man who distributes blessings through his psychotic talk, but who still comes every month to the clinic, to receive his phenothiazine injection. I have learned to value the real meaning of goodness and beauty behind the ugly man. I have learned to value limping Sa'adia coming to the clinic breathing heavily and puffing up the hill. I have especially learned to understand that even a disease can bring redemption, salvation, and health.

Andre, hi,

It is a beautiful summer's day outside, not too hot, with a slight breeze coming in from the sea. I feel very much at ease within myself. So, it was just the right time for me to tell you that it is so well described and sensitively written. I could almost see Sa'adia walking up the hill and yourself with your doctor's case full of miracle cures, both walking up that same hill together. You are such a good hearted and old family doctor, reminding me of the one that came to treat my family and myself in my youth. I must admit that I almost shed a tear when reading your vignette!

Love,

Stan

CHAPTER 10

The wonderment of strength

Stanley Rabin

As time goes on in my psychotherapeutic experience of the past 32 years, I cannot but marvel at the inner resources and strengths of some of my patients and its effect on me. After more than three decades of psychotherapeutic experience, I often feel humble in their presence. I think of my very fortunate position whereby clients share their innermost narratives with me, and I remind myself of my good fortune.

Jody, a 47-year-old happily married mother of two, a 23-year-old son and an 18-year-old daughter, was one of them. Jody was a senior high-tech worker who came to see me because of a peculiar, constant tingling sensation in her throat, which made it difficult for her to swallow. In the past there was a suspicion of esophagus obstruction. She reported feelings of choking and nausea. She had intensive medical examinations and tests, all of which showed negative results. The diagnosis made was esophageal reflux. Yet all medication did not lead to any significant change in her condition, thus her referral for psychotherapy was a last-minute effort to release her from her pain.

Jody was also an opera singer, which made her case even more problematic. All these symptoms started after a ski trip to Switzerland three years earlier. Suddenly the weather changed and she found herself trapped with three other skiers in a severe snowstorm, and eventually they were rescued under very difficult conditions. She reported feelings of anxiety and fear. Jody felt petrified and hopeless. Another event took place at that time too. A very close cousin who had been ill for some time died. The news, which played constantly on her mind, was broken to her a few hours before her trip.

During our first sessions I tried to understand the experience of her symptoms, when they started and how long she had felt their intensity. Her attractiveness and her personality captivated me. She came across as a very socially involved, rather pedantic woman with somewhat rigid principles, yet very warm and caring. She often seemed very serious and I wondered what lay behind her somewhat controlled appearance. Of course the timing of her physical symptoms added to the mystery surrounding her. Over the weeks and then months of therapy we delved deeper into the trauma she had experienced on her skiing holiday and it was obvious that this event must have been the direct precipitant to her symptomatology – the fact that she felt trapped, helpless, alone and anxious. We also discussed her mourning over the death of her cousin, the possible guilt about her going on a skiing holiday notwithstanding her death, and that she did not attend her cousin's funeral.

With time, I began to understand other parts of her life narrative. I understood how her voice had played the major part in her survival. Her life story is as follows. Jody's parents were of Indian background. When Jody was a few months old, her 24-year-old father left her mother for another woman and Jody was cut off from her father until she temporarily reconnected with him at the age of 18 years, just prior to her army service in Israel. Her mother remarried and through this union four other half brothers and sisters were born. Jody's stepfather despised her. She was the modern Cinderella except that the young handsome prince was not always part of her story. The abuse she suffered was quite unbelievable. She was never allowed by him to eat at the same table as the family; she was made to do all the housework. Her stepfather physically abused her too. She was able to take a bath only once a week, when no one was around. Often she would be found walking the streets, sometimes begging for scraps of food and clothing from kind neighbors. Even on the Jewish holidays she was not allowed to sit around the family table. Her stepsiblings totally ignored her. Hearing her story made my hair stand on edge! How can it be that this woman sitting across from me was a successful professional, a happily married coping lady after suffering so much abuse, pain, rejection and deprivation?

Her story continues. She tells me that her inner voice spoke to her through-out her childhood and said that she would survive. When I tried to mention to her that she went through her own private holocaust she snapped at me and said that nothing can be compared to that terrible event and that my words were not appropriate. The interesting thing of course in her survival was her ability to talk, to ask for help even though she felt such shame. Somehow she also believed in her own self-worth. Self-worth? "What self-worth can anyone build up after being subjected to such extreme abuse?" I said to myself. During one particularly emotive session she suddenly wept and exclaimed: "This is the first time in my life that I have told my story. Neither my husband even nor of course my children know anything about my past. I didn't want to tell them." "Why?" I asked disbelievingly. "Because I don't want them or anyone else to feel sorry for me. Why should I subject them to so much pain?" she answered. I felt that just like among Holocaust survivors I was the only privileged person to hear her testament. I remember feeling very emotional at this stage. Her story continues.

At the age of 16 her mother, a simple and weak woman, herself abused by her husband, agreed that to keep "peace in the house" and maybe "to give me peace too," she would be sent to a boarding school on a kibbutz. Here came the turning point in her life. A 65-year-old woman, a Holocaust survivor, "adopted" her. "Yes," I thought, "it had to be one survivor who would recognize, understand, and care for another." She became very attached to the woman's family and adopted their culture. She sang in the local choir and this is when she developed her operatic talents, which she uses up to today. She as an excellent student bridged the gap in her studies and left the kibbutz to join the army as a person who functioned much better, and was more confident. In the military she flourished. She was regarded as a dependable, responsible, and capable soldier. She studied with the help of her adopted parents and got her degree in computer science. She made a brief contact with her biological father, was able to express her anger and revulsion towards him for abandoning her, and then cut off all contact with him.

She married Joseph, a supportive caring older man. The marriage was a very good one .She was also a good mother, able to shower her children with love yet knowing full well how to set limits. "Where, for God's sake," I asked myself, "did she get these maternal abilities when she was brought up (or brought down, more precisely!) by her totally abusive stepfather and her inadequate, passive mother?" Over the time in therapy, Jody learned the

Hi Stan,

Sometimes I wonder how much luck, just luck, we need in life. Jody had the luck to find a person that crossed her trajectory in life and for a time being they walked part of the road of life together. Both of them had a history of abuse and Jody was able to feel the pain of a Holocaust survivor and, through that, get some balance of her own suffering. Feeling compassion for the pain of the old woman, she learned to embrace and give solace to her own suffering in childhood, freeing herself from her own self-pity. As with many of the Holocaust survivors she also didn't want to talk about her suffering to the next generation; they can live on with an encapsulated trauma, not known by anyone, and the psychotherapist is in a special position to help these persons. In the sessions with you, you surely projected her strength and your belief in her ability to work through her suffering. In her childhood, she was not able to talk about her suffering, and you gave her this opportunity to express herself, to "clean" herself. In my experience of being a family doctor I also see patients with pain in their throat, strange sensations and difficulties in swallowing and very often this is a presentation of "irritable bowel syndrome," and more specifically a spasm in her pharynx. It is almost always related to anxiety symptoms, unknown inner feelings, repressed feelings that "want" to go out – to be shouted out – but they are choked, strangulated. This is where body and mind play together on the same stage and many physicians can learn from this case, expanding the anamnesis by exploring the patient's past history and suffering in life, and not seeing the symptoms solely through the gastroscopy tube.

Thanks for this opportunity.

Love,

Andre

CHAPTER 11

Intractable Michelle

Andre Matalon

I had a feeling of *déjà vu* when Michelle's psychologist called me yesterday to talk about her. Michelle is a very dependent patient of 32 years old, with a constant anxiety, panic attacks, irritable bowel syndrome, and pain all over – the dread of any family physician. Since the beginning of my relationship with her and her family I knew I would have great difficulty in caring for them. When they first transferred their files to me, it was about 17 years ago and Michelle was about 15 years old, the only child of a family who had emigrated from France. That's why it was so exciting for me, at the beginning. I was just a resident and it was nice to be chosen to be their family physician, especially talking to people in my mother tongue.

Michelle's grandmother was 80 years old, a Holocaust survivor who spoke terrible French with a Yiddish accent, and spoke no Hebrew at all; Michelle's mother was also her only daughter. Together, the three women represented the major bulk of visits to me, more so than any other family in my practice. All their visits would make me "dance" in my chair in obvious discomfort. I could understand that it was a dysfunctional family, but how could I work with them? They were always trying to find something wrong with my treatment and they continuously ask questions. "Why didn't you send her to hospital earlier?" "Why didn't you consider giving her new medicine for her diabetes?" "Why didn't you order a stool test for occult blood?"

After years of being afraid of their response I plucked up the courage and just asked them to search for another doctor, if they were so discontented with my caring and treatment and had so little confidence in my professional abilities. As I said this, I saw that they had become uncomfortable, and were moving restlessly in their chairs. From then on, I noticed a change in their attitude towards me. Each time that they began complaining, they would immediately search for different, more moderate words. This went on and on until the present time. Aging and diseases took over Michelle's parents' bodies. Meanwhile, Michelle married and gave birth, but still, her temper tantrums, frequent crying and emotional breakdowns were always accompanied by abdominal pain and visits to the emergency room. Three times Michelle has succeeded in beginning psychological treatment with a psychologist. Because she is clever, she can make initial connections but she is incapable of getting through more than five or six visits. In short, sometimes I think that she cannot make a real commitment except to me. Michelle is also almost dependent on Prozac, but she "doesn't like chemicals" and three to four months after beginning treatment she feels better, forgets to come for her medicines, and then finally stops treatment altogether.

Recently she had had difficulties in her workplace (she is a bank clerk) and again she was in distress and asked me for a referral for psychological treatment, "but this time it's for good, I promise I will adhere to treatment, I badly need it!" She finally wants to learn to treat herself through psychotherapy, and not be dependent all her life on Prozac, she claims.

But, yesterday, for me, was a turning point in our relationship. Her psychologist suddenly called me and informed me that she had already seen Michelle once a week for six consecutive weeks, and that Michelle had felt understood and her distress was less severe. However, the psychologist continued, Michelle had not come for her last two scheduled sessions. Her psychologist had tried to call her, but Michelle didn't answer her phone calls. Furthermore, Michelle had not paid her for any of the sessions. I was immediately overcome by guilt feelings, being the one who referred her. I felt bad and maybe also furious about Michelle's behavior, and thought seriously about discontinuing treating the family if they did not pay the therapist. Together with my anger and probably feelings of frustration I felt that I had some questions to ask myself as well: Have I the right to link my treating her to her continuing psychological intervention? May I do this? Am I also responsible for psychological treatment after the referral? I realized that I was being the paternalistic father, setting up clear demarcation lines for her, boundaries that were probably lacking in her upbringing. Setting boundaries may be the right thing for me to do for her, for her health and for her well-being, and it is probably the right thing for me as well! I was certainly setting boundaries for her by linking my treatment of her to her paying the psychologist. On the other hand I was interfering with financial matters, which are none of my business. But I then ask myself: What would happen if she doesn't want my limits? What are the limits of my responsibility in this case?

And what if she doesn't have sufficient resources and strength for psychological treatment?

Andre, hi,

About Michelle, I am now allowing my mind to "free associate" so if what I say does not directly touch you, please understand! In this case you seem to look at the limits of your responsibility, the boundaries we all set, or don't, for ourselves and our patients, and its inevitable impact on our professional lives, and ourselves. I try to keep up to the rules of boundary setting I learned in my early days, sometimes not so well as you will surely in the future see, when I write to you about the patient who never paid up!

Yet, as I become more mature in my professional life and more mature within myself, I have become more flexible and less demanding for ultimate professionalism. In your case, I feel that you may feel overly responsible for Michelle. Probably feelings of embarrassment too in that you were "responsible" for referring her to the psychologist but Michelle let you down, she cheated on you too, in a way. We often like to be appreciated by other professionals and when we 'let them down' (so to speak) it leaves us with ambivalent feelings. That's what happens to me anyway.

Another thought I had. We often take gleeful pride when other colleagues get manipulated. As if to say, it won't happen to me. I will be different! Yet I feel that you are concerned (understandably) by possibly being manipulated by Michelle. So you are right when you intimate that if Michelle has done this to the psychologist there is no guarantee that she will not do it to you too. I think that her behavior affects the most pinnacle cornerstone of our work as health professionals – the issue of trust!

Andre, I hope that this response of mine has helped you, as much as writing this down has helped me!

Warm regards,

Stanley

Dear Stan,

Thanks for your insights and your opening up new ways of looking at this case story. Now I feel that I was too harsh on her and maybe on myself. She is certainly ill and weak, even if she has just a personality problem. She herself is a victim of her upbringing. After your writing I was able to re-find a new compassion in supporting her.

Thanks,

Andre

CHAPTER 12

Paying for compassion

Stanley Rabin

A long time ago, in the twilight months of the last century, Joy was referred to me for therapy. Joy was in her mid forties, a mother of a 10-year-old daughter. She was physically healthy, but very depressed. She was in the throes of a very complicated and tumultuous divorce and had moved out of her home. Joy's father was in the chemical industry and was very successful. She was very attached to her father and dependent on him. She joined the family business, and as the company developed she was given more responsibility. Later she became the company director. However, the business eventually was forced to close down, because of government cutbacks. Joy was now financially troubled, with creditors continually threatening her. At this stage she became very anxious. Anxiety was soon replaced by depression, with symptoms of sadness, listlessness, weight loss, and sleeping problems becoming more and more evident. She devalues herself and there was suicidal ideation. This is when she consulted with me.

I saw Joy for about two years, during which there were times when she went into deep depression. Her worries were exacerbated by the stormy divorce, which came about when she learned that her husband was having an affair with her best friend. On occasion her husband called me, expressing his concern for her, even though they were getting divorced. Joy's father continued to support her initially, but recently he suffered a heart attack, and their relationship changed under the circumstances. I, of course, replaced the father and became more and more of a positive, supportive figure in Joy's life, playing this role gladly, as I was concerned with her welfare. At times she could not face her problems and stayed in bed all day. During this entire period she was given high doses of antidepressant medication, and this relieved some of her severe symptoms. Joy was dependent on our meetings and I realized that her very basic personality dependency needs had been transferred onto me. She often phoned me at home, and I would have lengthy discussions with her. She appeared to be a kind, sensitive woman, very much appreciative of my treatment.

Now comes the crux of my story. After about two years of psychotherapy, Joy slowly recovered from her depression, a result of the pharmacological treatment and my supportive involvement. Her wealthy brother set her up in a new business. Her divorce finally came through, and she later met a divorced man, and a loving and caring relationship developed. At this stage her depression had lifted and it was jointly decided that therapy should be terminated. She was still on a maintenance dosage of antidepressant medication, which stabilized her emotional state.

During the last year and a half in therapy when she was still severely depressed and needy, Joy's financial situation had reached a critical peak and one day she reported that she had no money to pay for her treatment. Moved by my compassion I took a very unconventional step and decided to allow her to pay whenever she could. So, for over a year I had been seeing Joy without taking fees. She seemed very touched by my gesture and so the months of treatment continued. After her recovery, when therapy was terminated, she promised to pay all the money she owed me. I was not worried (at this stage) about her intentions. However, months turned to a year, then three years had passed and I had heard not one word from her, neither about her progress nor about my money!

My feelings vacillated between feeling hurt and betrayed. Then I began to feel angry. Was Joy a charming engaging person, who set me up? I had been made to look a fool in my own eyes, when my compassion, concern and caring for her had been abused. I was now paying the price. It took me time to consider my next move. After further self-deliberation I wrote bills and mailed them to her. I called her at home, but never received an answer. Later, with my professional self-image damaged, I decided to turn to legal sources. My lawyer wrote a few legal letters but they were often returned stamped "address unknown." Time passed and my strong feelings were repressed or subsided as I readjusted my thinking, saying, "So you learn from your mistakes and this is a lesson you will not forget."

One morning I received a phone call from her. She was very disappointed by my lawyer's letters to her. She said that she is still in dire economic distress and my request just added to her desperate state. I tried my best to "act the businessman," but as the conversation progressed I suddenly found myself on the defensive. I pointed out that in over three years I had not even heard from her until now.

"You were the person I trusted most in the world and now you are letting me down," she exclaimed. Has she emotionally entrapped me again? I began to feel remorse and guilt that I had even contacted her, demanding my debt! Maybe I had been too hard on her? Will I succumb? Well, I did! My psychotherapeutic heart overcame me again. I would trust her just once more. I agreed to temporarily withdraw the legal procedures, and contacted my lawyer who sent her a summary of our agreement pointing out that she should start paying off her heavy bill to me forthwith.

This case left me confused. Did I have the right to start legal proceedings due to nonpayment of therapy bills in an emotionally disturbed patient? What happens when trust is shaken in the psychotherapeutic alliance? Can one continue treating patients who have abused our trust? What happens when money interferes with our relationship with patients? How should we act "appropriately"? What price do we pay for our compassion? Somehow I comfort myself and take solace in the fact that even after the price I had paid for my compassion (I have since received part of my due payment), I treasure my belief in the basic goodness of man.

Hi Stan,

This case is very interesting, touching and sad . . .

Now about the name of this narrative – I think it says it all – "The price of compassion." You don't have to add the word "monetary."

Andre

Dear Andre,

Yes, you have made a relevant point here. It is not only monetary compassion that is worrying me but compassion generally. I now see I must find compassion also in being able to forgive myself – for making such an obvious mistake, by not being professional enough. I preach this to my students in supervision every week but here I go right ahead and make the same damn mistake!

Rethinking the case, I now see that, while I treated Joy for so long without getting financial compensation, I am sure that I received emotional compensation in helping her without limits, probably related to my own need to be needed, and need to please, and to be omnipotent!

Shalom,

Stanley

CHAPTER 13

On feeling offended

Andre Matalon

I have been treating a particular family for over 20 years. The grandmother, Lea, about 82 years old, is an old lady who suffers mainly from Parkinson's disease, and also from hypertension, glaucoma, ischemic heart disease and arthritis. Last year I also diagnosed senile dementia and she then went to live with her only son and had a Philippine nurse assistant. She is bed ridden, but just sits sometimes in front of the TV. She always complains that she doesn't feel good, and over the last five years I've made home visits once every two to three months. Our relationship was almost perfect – I was the kind, ideal, and noble visiting doctor, who does not take money for visits. I also had a good relationship with her only son, an officer in the police force, and we always spoke freely and with kinship feelings, when I visited his mother.

One year later, Lea lost control of her sphincters and the last visits were less and less agreeable to me. I felt myself rejecting the family requests for home visits, but to no avail – I found myself visiting her more and more, sometimes more than once a month. There was always another request for a home visit, because of "severe" problems or serious causes – syncope, fever and so on. I spoke to her son and asked him to consider transferring her to an old-age home, but he gently turned down my suggestion.

Last week I was called again to make a home visit, after Lea had apparently lost consciousness. Instinctively I didn't want to go, because I was there three days before. Over the phone I heard that she was already feeling better, so after offering a referral to the emergency room which was refused by the family, I ordered blood tests. I thought that it could be a brain tumor or a transient ischemic brain attack. I ordered the blood tests but I forgot to call the nurse to make a home visit. The next day, at 8:10, there was a frustrated telephone call from Lea's son, who said that nobody came to visit his mother and how could I have forgotten to talk to the nurse? I immediately turned to the nurse and she went to Lea's house to take the blood tests, which were all normal. Lea's condition was exactly the same as it was before.

But, for some few days after then, something was broken in my heart. I felt rejected and offended, after all I had done for her and her family! Even knowing that the son was probably displacing his anger and helplessness at his mother's brain damage and Alzheimer's onto me, I still felt hurt. Then I suddenly had an insight that I was, myself, maybe displacing some frustration in losing my "ideal doctor" fantasy that I was trapped in.

Now, months after this incident, I can feel again in me those known feelings of love and kinship for this family and admire the son's efforts and love towards his very sick mother.

Dear Andre,

Our profession is one of caring and healing and treating. Sometimes this can be with overwhelming and unrealistic demands.

We try to please, to give the best that we can, and most often we are appreciated. But when suddenly we feel the rage or the frustration of the patient or the family, all our psychological defenses are let down. Even though we can understand that our patient may be displacing his anger and pain onto us, this understanding is sometimes not enough. It stays on the intellectual level, and our feelings of being rejected are on an emotional level that must be attended to.

Maybe by you writing to me you can integrate both levels of your reaction.

Yours,

Stan

CHAPTER 14

Abuse, freedom, and me

Stanley Rabin

Dana was a 46-year-old woman who came to see me after being referred by her husband David, a colleague physician. David thought that she needed help because of her continual headaches, possible anxiety-related hypertension, and "her recently suspicious behavior." I was sitting quite eagerly waiting to receive this special patient whose husband had a very senior post and was an important figure in the regional general hospital. So when Dana appeared I was surprised to see a petite, dark, attractive-looking woman who looked much younger than her age. She was courteous and pleasant in her manner and was very forthcoming with her responses to my questions.

Her general background immediately intrigued me. She was born in South Africa (my birthplace too). Her family was of Indian descent; she was classified in Old South Africa as a "nonwhite woman," and was brought up in a nonwhite section of Cape Town. At the age of 19 years Dana eloped with David, a white Jewish South African. The couple went to the UK and married there. Three years after David's specialization, the family immigrated to Israel on David's initiation. The move to Israel was of course not easy. Further inquiries revealed the following background facts. Her three siblings (she was the youngest of two sisters and two brothers) were brought up by her hardworking and dedicated mother while her abusive father was either drinking with his friends or philandering with other woman. Dana was exposed to a great deal of tension between her parents in which her father was emotionally (and on rare occasions physically) abusive towards his wife. Dana then gave me an account of her relationship with David. She told me of their marriage, her conversion to Judaism, his successful medical studies and his career. She told me about David with much pride, yet I sensed in her a bit of sadness. This feeling became even more pronounced when she let me into the secret world of their marriage. David had been emotionally abusive to her. Her doting over him delighted him. He was very controlling, insisting to know her every move. He himself never missed an opportunity to flirt with other women. He would touch them in her company, invite them sometimes to their home without her permission, and then ask them to work out with them in their workout room. A lot of touching took place, with Dana being the passive observer. David criticized her work ability even though she was well established as a senior programmer in a high-tech firm. Rumors were heard of David's encounters with nurses in the hospital but David would deny this when hesitantly questioned by Dana.

It was clear to me that Dana was in a replicate marriage of her parents' relationship. She was using blanket denial to cover up her fears and I was aware that I had to carefully allow her to look into these fears. During the first meetings she was convinced that she was "overly exaggerating my fears" and was not sure that there was any reason to come to see me. I realized that keeping her in therapy was important, and also that I should be careful that she not become overly dependent on me. However, I had my own fears about my attachment to Dana, as I became more and more entranced by her story. I was suddenly flooded by my own long forgotten personal memories. Firstly I became very much enchanted by her background, especially since, unlike me, she was raised on "the other side of the apartheid fence." My story with the apartheid regime was mixed. I got my professional training in South Africa yet despised the system. However, my political involvement then was minimal, as was that of my white leftist intellectual friends. Secondly, I was aware that my eagerness to cure Dana was somewhat linked to my long repressed wish to ease my own conscience, to finally put things right for myself. I felt that having been a privileged white South African I myself had abused the system and the "nonwhites." Thirdly, her beauty, her sensitivity, her intelligence and her gracious femininity mesmerized me. For all these reasons I realized the importance of going easy and keeping clear boundaries. With this in mind I got to work!

Dana revealed to me that her thoughts of being betrayed were slowly getting the better of her. Careful examination ruled out paranoid ideation. Dana told me of her devotion and loyalty to her husband and her total idealization of him. Yet she reported her husband's involvement with other woman, his "lovey dovey" touching and seducing women in her presence and her general repugnance of this behavior. At the same time she felt too scared to confront him, lest he be angry with her and then reject her. During our sessions Dana recounted her mother's devotion to her father and his emotional abuse of her. She slowly understood the connection between her parents' behavior and her own. For the first time in her life she then expressed some anger towards David. He, of course, was angered by her assertiveness, which threatened the delicate balance of their relationship.

At this stage I used a term familiar and appropriate for both Dana and myself. The magic word was empowerment. I recounted how much she was disempowered in apartheid South Africa and that on a more personal micro-level she made herself disempowered in her marriage. She doted on her husband without limits, discarding her own self-worth and her true self. Her own self had slowly slipped away. She constantly mirrored herself through him, and became intertwined, enmeshed within the narcissistic self of her husband. She began to disentangle herself from him, and was able to look into herself, a process involving much fear, pain, and sadness. For years she had capitulated to aggressive men, starting with her own father when she protected and identified with her submissive mother, and then her husband. Slowly she was able to reach individuation; she began to realize her own needs, desires, and wishes, and accepted her own self-worth. As our talks progressed there was a general improvement in her physical condition as she gained insight into herself. She expressed to me the difficulties she had in expressing angry feelings generally and to David in particular, and her fears of rejection should she become more assertive in the marriage, and her constant need to be accepted and liked.

Dana's abusive narrative and its repair through therapy became quite clear to me. She had the insight to realize her abusive relationship, the masochistic element she was playing in it and the need for her to break the family generational circle of female abuse. We later spoke of her improving relationships with male figures generally. At work she was now able to express herself to her male boss and assert her rights. She was also able to accept the positive feedback that she received at work and from her friends who generally adored her positive disposition. She realized that it was important for David and for her to go for marital therapy and she put it to him one evening. He then "spilt the beans." He admitted to her that over the past year he was having an intense love affair with one of the nurses on the ward. He stated that he "still loved her," and asked her to be understanding, forgiving, and accept the other woman. Dana was shocked but somehow relieved. Her suspicions were well founded. Her husband's insistence for her to come to see me was "to make me crazy when in fact my suspicions were correct." She felt deceived by David's insistence that she come for therapy, and also felt she had gained so much from our sessions. Her anger slowly decreased as she reached resignation and acceptance. She felt she had personally grown over the months.

Dana now made her decision. She decided to separate from David, notwithstanding his pleas for her not to do so. After this decision David made one final request. He begged her not to tell their friends of the real reason for her leaving him (the affair) since he felt it would undermine his professional and personal image in the community. She realized that even now he wanted to control her; she chuckled quietly to herself and flatly refused. She left him, and moved to another city where she was able to lead an independent life, carefully assessing her relationship with men so as not to get into a dependent, abusive and addictive relationship again as we had discussed in our therapy sessions. And for me? Her story took me down paths I never liked to confront in myself. Through my repairing Dana's story, I was repairing my own story. I realized that by empowering Dana I was also freeing myself of my own shackles of frustration, pain, guilt of being a privileged white South African abusing the underprivileged others for my own comfort and advancement. By freeing Dana I was able then to finally free myself. I asked myself many questions. Was I helping Dana for my own needs or for hers? Did I covertly disclose my conflicts to her? Did I subtly push her to divorce David? I remember realizing the intensity of my feelings and my wish to keep reacting empathically to her, yet to keep my boundaries by not becoming too emotionally overloaded or coldly professional. Had I succeeded in disengaging our stories?

At our last meeting Dana expressed her appreciation for the sessions. She said that she would always remember the words that were spoken and the feelings they had aroused in her. She stated that her decision to leave David was the first real decision she had made for herself. I felt relieved. She felt ready to be tested in any next future encounter with men. "I now finally know the danger signs," she said.

This last meeting was close to the Passover Festival so I decided to tell Dana another story, a story known to us both, the Biblical story of Passover. I then said to her, "Just as the children of Israel went out of Egypt from slavery to freedom so you yourself have over the past months done. You have freed yourself from your own personal bondage." This was not an easy thing for me to say because I was aware that I was talking to myself too. So as I slowly looked up I noticed that tears were rolling down her cheeks – and mine! We shed our tears, and dried our eyes as I shook her hand and bade her a very warm and fond goodbye.

Dear Stan,

Dana reminds me of the case story I wrote to you some months ago, "intractable Michelle." She spoke my mother tongue; she shared a common culture and conflicts. But there was a difference in that Dana was also very attractive as you mentioned, and it took me back to the "girl of Ipanema." I could feel through your narrative a combination of the passion, the forbidden, the untouchable and unattainable. Maybe you felt the same?

What do you think, Stan?

Andre

Hi Andre,

You certainly aroused old feelings in me. In the apartheid of South Africa where we grew up, even liberals like me were curious about the colored women, the black, there were feelings of enticement and mystery in what would happen if we "went over the line." This filled us with curiosity but was dangerous then. Another point that struck me, relating to the way I view color. Even today I must shamefully admit that I automatically classify people into the color of their skins, and then feel so much anger and guilt all at the same time. Anger, at that cruel system in which I grew up, which, even after all these years, still manages to taint my very soul. Guilt, about which I have not yet found the way to free myself. So as you see your point triggered off a lot of associations in me.

Regards,

Stan

CHAPTER 15

The helper's helplessness: Enrique's story

Andre Matalon

I was depressed when I got home from my last house call. After 20 years of practicing medicine it is not often I feel helpless, at least not to the point of shaking my mental equilibrium. I thought that writing this story and sharing it with you could lighten my burden.

Enrique was born in Argentina. Now 75, he is married and childless. He has lived in Israel for 35 years, the last 20 in retirement following myocardial infarction and bypass surgery. Since childhood, disease and death had overshadowed his life. Enrique is the youngest of 10 siblings, five of whom died in childhood of unknown causes. Another brother died of a heart attack at age 33. Enrique's father also died of a heart attack when Enrique was an adolescent, and he remained with his mother who died of cancer when he was 37, and he himself nursed her through her illness to her death. He describes her as a bitter, domineering woman who was highly critical of others and would not accept any criticism herself.

Enrique was a textile worker. After his mother's death, overwhelmed with loneliness, he decided to immigrate to Israel, and it was on the sea voyage to Israel that he met his future wife. In Israel he worked in the textile industry, a job he did not enjoy. His low wages forced his wife to seek work caring for children, and one of these children was our firstborn son. We were neighbors, I was then a medical student, also an immigrant from South America, and Enrique used to call on me in the evenings to seek my advice on simple matters. He even consulted with me about undergoing bypass surgery following myocardial infarction, a prospect that scared him very much. I felt honored, even flattered, that he consulted with me. Perhaps I was a substitute for the son he didn't have, with him and his wife acting as "grandparents" raising my first child. But he was also a nervous, bitter, and complaining person, very different from my life-loving father. When I became a family physician at the local clinic, Enrique and his wife promptly joined my list of patients.

Life treated him harshly. During his 15 years as my patient he was hospitalized repeatedly for chest pains. While most of these episodes were musculoskeletal, he had also undergone cardiac catheterization and PTCA (percutaneous transluminal coronary angioplasty). He also suffered from headaches, a sensation of burning on his tongue, pains in his eyes, upper abdominal pains, and backaches, and his life gradually contracted into doctor visits, treatments, and hospitalizations. Enrique no longer prepared asado on Saturdays and rarely visited the few friends who were still willing to listen to his "Adventures in Medicine Land."

Health fund regulations allowed him to see specialists without referral from the family physician. This served his basic problem – somatization – the last barrier before his total depression. Despite our years of contact and my improving communication skills, Enrique was unable to make the mind–body connection. We talked about life, about the cancer that was discovered in his brother, his sister's death and even about the loss of his libido and potency. We discussed the "golden years," the hypocritical euphemism for the ongoing suffering of old age. We discussed serotonin and Prozac. Any antidepressive medication he took always brought about "severe" side effects. Although he was closely monitored and often saw me twice a week, he was unable to endure the initial period of adjustment to new medications, perhaps also refusing to see himself as what he pejoratively termed "mentally ill." He would cunningly appear with a letter from a neurologist who would recommend discontinuing the medication while requesting additional tests.

In retrospect I feel that I was in coalition with his wife, a domineering and realistic woman, who angrily and grudgingly assumed the role of caretaker.

She accepted my referral to counseling at the mental health clinic, if only to learn to reduce the tension between them. Quite possibly, this coalition could have increased his feeling of rejection and served as the ultimate proof that he was misunderstood.

During a particularly difficult period following rehospitalization in the neurological ward for examining the source of his headaches, the doctors suggested psychiatric counseling. He consented to day-care treatment in a psychiatric hospital; partly because of my "aggressive" determination – for which I have no regrets – that psychiatric treatment should be a condition for me to carry on treating him.

Enrique agreed to be hospitalized for a trial period of a few weeks. These stretched to almost a year, the best year since his retirement. Enrique, the psychiatric team, and I agreed that he would see specialists only after consulting with me and after I had approved a given test. A few months later I came to visit Enrique at the psychiatric ward and found him acting as the foreman in the occupational therapy workshop, as well as a "father" to young people with schizophrenia.

His condition improved, and he had to be released. On the evening preceding his release an ambulance was called to his home, and Enrique was hospitalized in ICU (intensive care unit) with recurrent myocardial infarction. This time the infarct was accompanied by cardiac failure. The following cardiac catheterization ended in a severe stroke, rendering Enrique incapable of speaking and weak in the right side of his body. Six weeks later he was transferred for rehabilitation to a local day-care facility. Here again he felt secure, surrounded by doctors and nurses, and functioned to the outmost of his physical abilities. Again, improvement meant release.

Enrique is back home now. His speech is impaired. Each sentence rolls heavily on his tongue, and his impatience with himself brings him to immediate tears and choking. He cannot eat, shave, or take a shower independently, but is capable of getting up and walking around without a cane. By law he is entitled to three hours of help five days a week, which he reluctantly accepts, though he spends most of his time in bed. Despite his reluctance, this assistance allows his wife some breathing space.

Enrique wants to die. His attending psychiatrist changed his antidepressants again, and since he cannot speak, he cannot benefit from psychological counseling – which he does not want anyway.

Enrique is a wise man. He understands everything happening to him and around him, but is interested in nothing. Even soccer no longer holds his attention. He suffers maddening, inexplicable pains, and continues his years-long habit of taking several daily doses of over-the-counter analgesics. When his wife leaves for work he cries bitterly, begging her not to go. The ambulatory cardiac emergency service has warned Enrique that they will stop responding to his almost daily calls. The hospital no longer admits him when he is brought to the emergency room, and the cardiologist is angry with him whenever he sees him, partly out of anger with his own inability to help. When I call on him, I detect in myself more anger than compassion. I am angry with a person who does not want to help himself. Next, I feel guilty. How can I be angry with a person who is in such agony? How can I be angry at a person who suffers disease and depression that prevent him from any rational discourse on life, impair his ability to enjoy himself, and destroy any positive feelings? Frustrated by my inability to get through to him, I am also frustrated by my inability to look creatively into my bag of tricks and pull out a new potion or magic that will rekindle my desire to treat him.

This time I prescribed opioids, hoping they will succeed where communication, caring, commitment, and devotion failed. He is "blinded" by headaches, abdominal pains, and chest pains, which he claims are the sole source of his suffering. I tell him to wait until the current antidepressant begins to help. But, equally "blinded" by my helplessness, I no longer believe my own words.

Epilogue

Writing to you proved beneficial to me, Stan. When we talked about him, last week in my car, you pointed out aspects of Enrique's personality that I had failed to notice. I remember you talking about him as a bottomless pit, as a tragic figure, with an abysmal deprivation that could not ever be fulfilled. Enrique needs all his caregivers, depending on us to help in his endless quest for something to fill this void, yet he frustrates us. He frustrates us in that very special place, our need to give, to help, to heal, and perhaps even to love. All entries to him are blocked. He is the typical dependent clinger who turns into a help rejecter, a trait that family physicians always find very difficult to deal with. Indeed, a major part of my frustration was caused by Enrique's rejection of my helping hand, which is my mainstay and stock in trade, and without which I feel worthless. This is especially poignant in the case of depression, as I have always been "Andre the Warrior Against Depression," a role that I have played since I was eight years old and already knew I wanted to be a doctor. The counter-transference makes it clear that Enrique frustrates me in my inability to help him, throwing me back to my known childhood feelings of impotence and helplessness at my mother's depression. This may be the reason I found it difficult "just to be there" without "doing" anything. I kept on imagining that admission to any type of treatment facility would help him again.

Talking to you, Stan, I understood that my feelings – anger, frustration, depression, and helplessness – could also possibly be Enrique's. It seems that Enrique transfers onto his caregivers all his helplessness and anger at his mother who was never capable of loving him after the death of his older siblings. These feelings were transferred to me in such a way that I, too, felt them, in a process that you, psychologists, call projective identification. Enrique lives in monumental fear, actually terror, of death, yet at the same time wants it. Only when hospitalized, when he felt constantly embraced by the presence of doctors and nurses, did his fear of death subside and he felt better.

Some of my medical colleagues pointed out the severity of his illness, so severe that cardiologists and neurologists determined that there was nothing more they could do to save him, and only I, the family doctor, maintained a fantasy of omnipotence. Furthermore, I had to let go of another one of my fantasies, the one in which all my patients will reach their end having "accepted" death. Sadly, there are some, and herein lies Enrique's tragedy, that will arrive at death in bitterness and anger.

The solution to this feeling of helplessness was then the collaboration with you. Looking at the patient's feelings, while also looking at my own, provided me with a feeling of growth and personal and professional development.

For these I am grateful to you, and to Enrique. Thank you, Enrique. I am now able to be there with you.

I visited Enrique after our talk and changes of ideas. I now felt differ-ently about him and equipped with greater understanding of his condition. This visit was not another in a chain of predictable frustrations, and I felt, following the processing, that I could let go of my need to be the savior. The opioid hadn't done much good. However, our talk took a new direction when I was able to turn to his wife and mirror her anger towards him, which was, just like mine, a part of Enrique's anger with his condition. It was then that he began crying, and so did she and I felt meaning and sense of coherence returning to me. Blurry with tears I could now see new space for work, and could share Enrique's grief for a life spent in the shadow of death.

Dear Andre,

I am very happy that I was part of the help that allowed you to reframe his story, and your own. Thank you for the confidence in me and for the opportunity you gave me to be with you in this difficult case.

All the best,

Stan.

CHAPTER 16

Psychotherapy without talking

Stanley Rabin

This week, George, a 55-year high-tech director, completed a year of psychotherapy with me. He was handicapped after suffering from a CVA (cardiovascular accident) a year and a half previously. We were in the process of terminating therapy, which provided me with the perspective of considering his gains and mine. George's left arm and leg had improved, and although his speech was still very deficient, he told me that he felt less dependent on others. During the course of our meetings, almost without words, he explained to me that I helped him to regain control over his life. It was only when we spoke in simple terms about his prognosis that he understood the essence of his state. This made it possible for him to internalize his predicament, emotionally come to terms with his loss and then move on the road to acceptance and resignation. In George's case, talking, although limited, was still the medium of choice, very different from Barry, another patient I treated a few months back.

Barry was a married 45-year-old accountant, father of two, who was run over by a car while crossing the road at a pedestrian crossing. He was injured, in a coma for three weeks, brain damaged with emotional and cognitive dysfunction. He was severely handicapped, not being able to walk, both feet and arms paralyzed and he was not able to speak at all. In fact, he was only able to vaguely grunt out the words, which often frustrated the medical personnel who attended him. Because of the inability to communicate with him, he was conveniently considered as being much more brain damaged than he actually turned out to be. Barry's source of strength was his devoted wife who tirelessly and uncompromisingly supported and encouraged him. I had already gotten puzzled frowns from the head health professional of the HMO (health maintenance organization) for agreeing to see him for psychotherapy. Was I crazy? I felt she was saying – what therapy could one offer to a brain-damaged individual who could just about grunt out his words? Was I a psychotherapist or a glorified baby sitter, she was probably saying to herself.

But I took up the challenge.

I decided at first that Barry would try and verbally express himself to me but when we became increasingly frustrated at his inability to communicate properly we decided jointly that he would write down on a computer what he was thinking and I would answer him verbally. This turned out to be a good choice at first though obviously a time-consuming and tedious encounter. Later on he acquired a laptop, which made things easier. Be the limitations as they were, throughout our close relationship I was captivated by his warm personality, his intelligence, and, most importantly, by his wonderful sense of humor. He would often crack a joke and even had the audacity to laugh about me, at my expense! His laugh was an infectious, loud, delightful growl and, when he laughed, his whole face lightened up. What was even more apparent was the communication he showed through his expressive eyes, which were my point of communication with him.

There were times of obvious sadness too as he explained to me the scope of his loss, his doubts and fears for the future, his loneliness, the depth of his misery, his struggle to find ways to readjust on the long road ahead. He wrote about suicide once, yet with his infectious smile and twinkle in his eyes, he reassured me that day that these were only thoughts, since "Relax, Doc! How the hell do you expect me to do it, being the wreck I am?" We wrote a lot. So many sensitive areas were discussed, as we touched each other's souls. Barry has over the years taught me much about coping, of the hardiness of the soul but more importantly the way one can in all adversities appreciate and adapt to life under the most difficult challenges. This was much more than talking psychotherapy in the conventional sense. It was a case of a different sort of psychotherapy, which induces the therapist and patient to be jointly involved, integrating different modes of communication and treatment modes. Barry allowed me to learn how to be a different therapist, finding in myself creative means for communication. Through him and his bold approach towards his handicap I also was able to understand the very essence of human fortitude, grace and coping, the very meaning of life. I was also able to appreciate and admire his loving and dedicated wife, constantly engaged in his treatment and rehabilitating process. Barry was also a caring and devoted father to his two children. They, too, learned to understand his warmth and affection expressed to them in a nonverbal mode of communication.

I think of the satisfaction we receive from treating such patients. The routine of clinical practice can be very tiring and monotonous. We see the same catastrophic ideations in the panic attack victim, or involve ourselves in the frustrating details of the obsessive-compulsive patient with whom we have so much sympathy, but whose ruminations make their lives difficult. This is why one of the most gratifying moments for me, as a practicing clinician, is to find pleasure in the way some of my patients, like George and Barry, present their life narratives, and how they have learned to cope so nobly with their suffering.

Hi Stan,

I am more accustomed to treating people with disabilities, including old persons after CVA with severe speech impairment and sometimes also new immigrants who do not speak any of the languages I know. These cases are very challenging but can also be very frustrating. In these cases we develop all our senses to understand their suffering and to join with it. It is really different from the traditional "talking cure" of the psychologists. We develop our observational senses, looking at body language, facial expressions, tone of voice, and the music underneath the content. There is also an international "code" in family practice. People like to be checked and touched; it makes them feel understood. By checking their bodies when a symptom is presented, people feel understood and maybe this is unique to family medicine – the integration aspects of body and mind. Your patient and your therapy reminded me of my own setting. It was indeed a different sort of psychotherapy where you had to be at your best to make room for creativity and courage. You also praised these two men's strength. By doing this you helped them to reconstruct their stories in a more functional way. You were there for them, you accepted their limitations and handicap and, by doing so, they were able to find inside themselves the alternatives for a better coping and living.

Love,

Andre

Dear Andre,

Thanks for the comments. You are right. Maybe it is important to show that psychotherapy does not only have to be practiced using the talking code. In Barry's case I looked at nonverbal signs, like his eyes. We also communicated with pen and paper, through his laptop, and later through email and other means. Maybe this shows the possible different and changing modes of communication in psychotherapy.

Keep cool. I hope you are enjoying the writing as much as I am!

Have a great week.

Stan

CHAPTER 17

Late understandings on death and love

Andre Matalon

Roszika was a 55-year-old Hungarian woman. When I first met her she had lived in Israel for many years, and was married and a mother of a 15-year-old daughter, and a 19-year-old soldier. I was then a 30-year-old recently graduated doctor, just beginning my specialization in family medicine. She held a doctorate in German literature, and was a poet and translator, an extremely intelligent and interesting woman. Her brightness and charisma overshadowed her handicap – she had a severe chronic lung disease caused by tuberculosis that she had suffered when she was a child in the concentration camps. Her breathing was all sound – loud, harsh, and frightening breath sounds, a result of her lung disease. Her health and life difficulties were many but she found comfort and support in her beautiful daughter. Anna was a tall, loving and helpful adolescent. Her beauty radiated, in marked contrast with the heavy, somber, dark furniture and general atmosphere of their house. I almost didn't see her son. But at this time, Roszika's greater difficulty was not her health, but nursing her husband.

Most of our encounters took place at their house, when I was called to treat her husband Kurt, 20 years her senior, suffering from Alzheimer's disease. He had frequent coughs from food aspirations, several episodes of fever and delirium, and urinary tract infections. He could not even walk alone. As a new doctor my first impressions were that through treating him I would become skilled at dealing with difficult symptoms, without the technologies that I had learned to rely upon during my medical training. Each time I had suggested it, the family refused to take him to hospital. The only time they complied was after he fell with an obvious fracture of the femur neck, and they just could not keep him standing up any more.

At the hospital, following the family's repeated efforts to get him on his feet, he received blood transfusions because of internal bleeding. Unfortunately after his fall, his cognitive functions further deteriorated and the doctors decided not to operate on him since he would not be an appropriate candidate for rehabilitation. He was then confined to bed, as any movement would generate great pain. A few days later pressure sores developed and the family was informed of the doctors' wish to transfer him to a nursing home. After a family discussion they decided to take him home and nurse him by themselves. He became a living vegetable, without human perceptions, feelings, or recognition of others.

I was suddenly involved in a treatment that I was not prepared for – home hospitalization. The pressure sores were already very deep and large and in less than a month he would hardly eat any food, in his state of semi-stupor. The family, with the agreement and blessing of my tutor, their long-standing personal family physician, accepted the inevitable and prepared for his death. He wished to die at home, in his own bed, and mentioned this frequently over the previous 10 years. The family also decided not to feed him by a gastric tube.

The next 10 days were the most difficult of my medical life, as my tutor had requested that I follow him up. At the end of my working day, I would come to their house, either to examine him or to talk to Roszika and Anna. Most of our discussions involved death and dying, especially the different philosophical approaches toward dying. I was directed by my tutor to read *On Death and Dying* by Elisabeth Kubler-Ross, an American psychiatrist who interviewed dying patients. Anna would escape from most of our common meetings, but at that time I lacked the understanding and maturity required to be aware of her suffering. I was overwhelmed by my own feelings. I remember well my fear and apprehension each time I had to go for the home visits. It was almost as if I myself was passing through all the stages described in the book. I would often come home depressed, sometimes angry at what I had experienced. But Roszika was always there, talking to me, reassuring me that we were doing the right thing. She even went to her books and brought to me papers on different views and significance of death in the literature. She paid special attention to the Buddhist philosophy of "good death," while dealing with and rejecting the accusations of some of her family members who felt that she was treating her husband cruelly. I went to their house every day for 10 days, each day thinking that this would my last visit, but it went on and on. His body was getting thinner and thinner, and his breathing became more and more shallow. Roszika and Anna changed places at his bedside every eight hours, washing and cleaning him up and preparing him for his last breath. I kept on thinking of their courage all the time. I failed to get them out of my mind, yet I had an inner feeling of calm, respect and being part of an important life lesson. I did not understand all its implications then. I also could not believe it would last so long. After 10 painful days, Kurt died. I was, of course, there to be with them and signed all the formalities for the burial. I decided not to go to the funeral but, again, I was there the same evening for the family gathering of the Jewish shivah, the ritual seven days of mourning during which people call on the family to comfort them. The ambience was cold and correct, but by my coming the atmosphere changed, and I could immediately feel their love and gratitude. Inside myself, I felt that it was me that should be sitting there – I had to mourn not only for my lost innocence in treating my first dying patient, but also for the re-discovery of my own deep fear of dying.

Time went by and I lost contact with the family. I once recognized Anna at an art fair. She told me that she dropped out of formal education, made her life as an artist and went to live in a boat in another city. She was even more beautiful, a young frightened adolescent. She also informed me that her mother was getting old and sick.

Suddenly, 15 years later, Roszika came back into my life again. She got my telephone number and invited me for a house call. I was quite apprehensive at the beginning. All sorts of feelings from the past reawakened in me. Why was she calling me? It took no time for me to learn that she herself was now dying and wanted my help and assistance in her dying. She told me that she remembered my understanding and sensitivity when dealing with her husband's disease and dying. She had just been released from hospitalization for respiratory insufficiency and had been on mechanically assisted ventilation for almost one month after a common cold. She was aware that a simple upper respiratory infection would deteriorate her respiratory functions again. She was definitely in agony, breathing through an oxygen mask, talking with extreme breathlessness, and with the same loud and frightening sounds of breathing that I would never forget. She had also "collected" more diseases. She now had a disabling tremor in her hands and was not able to write any more. She was also almost unable to read any more, because of her cataracts in both eyes and her fear of going through an operation. Each little change in her body, each simple viral infection, each change in her medications would immediately cause an exacerbation of her lung disease and she would be hospitalized with respiratory insufficiency for mechanical ventilation. She showed extreme difficulty in going through three hospitalizations in the last six months. She was alone at home, with a nurse visiting her for two hours a day, to help her with personal hygiene. Life for her was no longer worth living, as she was not able to read and write and did not have her children at her side. Roszika was not to change her children's decision and life trajectory. Her son was now a cellist in a German symphony orchestra and Anna lived 400 km from her. She asked me not to involve them in her condition and in her decision to end her life.

I was in an internal turmoil again. First of all I felt an understanding for Roszika's condition and existence. Secondly I felt a deep compassion for her. I remember the three hours sitting beside her, talking about her life narrative, her strength and determination to build a new life for herself after the Holocaust. She told me about her life with her husband, an older person, a "father-like" figure who loved her very much, but whom she respected more than loved. Then she surprised me by revealing another story. Her real love was expressed in a long secret affair with a married close friend. I was even more astonished when she disclosed his name – that of a person whom I had known very well. In my mixed feelings my mind wandered between two thoughts. Was it possible that it was her fantasy about the affair? I felt almost like a confessional priest taking her last vows and wishes. I understood that it was her secret life story that she was depositing in my "hands." She was preparing for her departure.

Along with my acceptance of her existential situation I also had angry feelings. She had called me to be her "executioner." I was inwardly frightened and in conflict. I could clearly feel my wish to run away. Fight or flight?

And, again, she was not asking me to take an active part in her death. She just asked me if any or all the drugs in her drawer were sufficient to kill her.

She couldn't accept the possibility of a failed attempt. How could or should I answer these direct questions? Was it right to take away all the drugs from her drawer? Was it necessary to hospitalize her, against her will, in a psychiatric hospital? But she was not at all delusional, not even depressed. Was it right for me to involve her children, against her will?

Now, five years later, I understand that she was not asking me which drug to take. She was intelligent enough to decide this for herself. With the insight I have today, I now realize that she simply was not able to die with her secret. In her wish to close her life with a clean slate and a clean conscience, she chose me to be her forgiver, the "confessional" priest/rabbi/doctor, to whom she had to reveal her secret. I also realize now that, in her death, she was still in love.

After writing this last phrase I felt a burst of tears. I realized some very important aspects of our personal and medical life that were present in this story: the right to die, the free will to decide about our own destiny, our right and privilege to participate in the most extreme situations of life, our role in guarding our dying patients' secrets, and being their ultimate conscience. All the doubts and dilemmas we have in our medical life were present in this story: what to do with our fears, courage, guilt, or shame. This story is also a mirror to each of us – it can happen to us. Will I be demented, will I lose all my humanity, will I suffer, will I be lonely at the end of life, will I have the internal strength to take decisions by myself or will there be somebody to listen to me? Is there "a good death"?

Maybe my burst of tears was related to our ultimate, total love that we want in our lives, and to die lovingly, filled with compassion. Suddenly I had a further flash of insight and things became clear for me: I was crying for my life being lived in the shadow of my own endless need and search for love.

Dear Andre,

I see the case as death anxiety, but also as pure love. Love that can never be realized in a formal, open way but is always a secret – maybe an exciting one, but one always locked up – to be shared only on the deathbed.

It is a story of death, courage, compassion, caring, and love.

Yes, as far as death is concerned, we all try to push it away until it creeps into our lives through the death of a friend, or a patient. Recently I experienced the death, a sudden unexpected death, of a patient of mine who shared his most intimate secrets with me – his secret lover, his love letters, and other very private information. Then it all just stopped – he had a heart attack while swimming in the sea and died . . . And all his personal and life secrets are now locked away for eternal safekeeping in my heart! It is as if everything stopped for him, and for me, at that critical moment!

I hope that this short note means something to you?

See you,

Stan

Stan,

It seems that relationships continue even after death – continuity – a cornerstone in Family Medicine.

I am still overwhelmed by the emotions this case brought to the surface – I was totally taken by Roszika these last days and I couldn't stop thinking about her.

Anyway – thanks for being there with me – I so much appreciate it.

I was not alone passing through my death anxiety!

Andre

CHAPTER 18

A time to reap and a time to change

Stanley Rabin

I have in my care a 38-year-old bachelor who has been in my treatment for a few years. During therapy he had a fleeting unstable relationship with a 43-year-old female professor in France whom he often visited when he studied at the Sorbonne for his MA in philosophy. When at home, he looked after his elderly parents, his father a UK-born architect, while his mother, French born, worked as a medical secretary. His mother had a serious stroke with complications and had been found recently to have colon cancer. Ron, the only child of this couple, had a very close relationship with his loving, caring and accepting mother and had a somewhat distant, but decidedly respectful relationship with his father. Ron presented to me as an intelligent, somewhat self-effacing, shy but very sensitive person. Throughout psychotherapy he had been trying to extricate himself from his parents' hold on him. Being an only child made this task particularly difficult. However, as therapy progressed, he was slowly able to take some concrete steps to become independent. He rented a flat with a close friend but then had to cope with loneliness and find ways to challenge his social anxiety.

At about the time of his mother's illness and her chemotherapy, Ron met Alice, a 30-year-old woman, a famous reporter who worked for a high-powered TV company. She was posted to Iraq and other Middle East stations and was soon promoted to chief regional reporter. It was at this time that Ron met her. He was infatuated by her good looks, her intelligence and her warm personality. He enjoyed their intimacy, and as time went on their relationship flourished and Alice became more and more significant for him. She would make short visits to Israel and on occasion they would meet in different countries. Because of her work, Alice had to make under-cover visits to Israel so all this romance was bound up in secrecy, with quick visits and hurried sex. However, the potential in the relationship was there and it was progressing fast! In the midst of this enveloping relationship Ron's mother died. This affected him greatly. Ron was left to cope with his own mourning and his father's intense grief. His father stopped working, and became acutely depressed, which required brief psychiatric intervention. Three months after his mother's death, I struggled to help Ron rebuild his life and to make him understanding of his grieving father. He also had to establish and build a new relationship with his father, but yet he had his own life to lead.

Yesterday he said something to me that affected me deeply. While he is now learning to cultivate his relationship with his father, he was enjoying his relationship with Alice. While Ron is helping his father to separate and disconnect from his late wife, he is now finally joining, connecting in his new relationship. He reported to me that while he is cuddling up, snuggling in bed with Alice, he sometimes thinks of his father sadly warming himself up alone, with blankets and bed covers and fond memories. "It is so ironic," he said. "While I am getting over my loneliness, my father is now being introduced to it."

I had a bit of a lump in my throat when he left me yesterday. I thought how the wheel of life turns, as someone reaps and someone has to learn to walk again. Especially now that in my life I am going through my own "rites of passage," learning to live with an empty nest as my children left home to live their own lives. With a tear in my eye, I think of the words of Pete Seeger's famous song from the sixties, "Turn, Turn, Turn . . .", adapted from the Bible:

To everything there is a season, and a time for every purpose, under
  heaven:
A time to be born, a time to die.
A time to plant, a time to reap.
A time to kill, a time to heal.
A time to laugh, a time to weep.

Hi Stan,

These last words of this song filled my heart with happiness. First of all, it is one of the best songs of "The Byrds" and I remember myself listening to this LP. It was in my mid-adolescent days, when I was struggling with my own separation-individuation tasks, struggling between following the American dream or the revolutionary path of social justice. Bob Dylan, Joan Baez and Che Guevara were my youth idols and, controversially, together with the semi-nude picture of Jane Fonda in *Barbarella*, they were all on the posters covering the walls of my bedroom. And now, fortunately after I have completed this task, I feel a sense of maturity and well-being. A sense of acceptance of the facts of life, acceptance of the life cycle, of your own unique passage through life, a sense of accomplishment, a sense of living a life with a time for every purpose, a time to laugh and a time to weep. You made me, I feel, more at peace with my past, with the child in me, a time to heal . . .!

Thanks, Stan.

Love,

Andre

Reflections and comments

Benyamin Maoz

After reading these narratives, I classified my impressions, associations, and reflections according to my own categories. Other readers may find different categories and subjects that appeal to them.

I tried to classify these reflections in certain passages to which I gave titles according to the main motive and idea, which each passage evokes in me. Now, I will describe my reflections in some detail.

Taking risks, quality of life (Narrative 1)

A family physician (GP) who evades treating difficult cases, referring every difficult patient to a specialist or to hospital, takes very few risks. Conversely, a family physician who dares to treat more difficult syndromes and diseases always takes a risk. Those who take risks may fail and may make mistakes. That should not happen too often, but it might. One should take personal and ethical responsibility for risks, mistakes and failures, even when the results are severe. There is a possibility that a reasonable, calculated but wrong decision may even cause death. If that happens one carries guilt feelings and secrets, which can be confessed only to a close and trustful person. Are quality of life and the patient's dignity important factors in medical decisions made today? Sometimes a therapist identifies with a patient, e.g. with an old man who lost control of his behavior and his personal dignity, while being hospitalized. Then we therapists think: Could it not happen to us? When shall we need hospitalization? After discharge from hospital, such a patient felt that he had "failed" in public, in hospital (what a shame!) and became depressed. Some physicians certainly take into consideration human factors, not only cold professional-technical ones. Just as their patients do, is it possible that physicians and therapists also wait sometimes for good luck and a miracle?

The wandering Jew (Narratives 2 and 18)

There are patients who have "a soul of an immigrant." During their lives they emigrated from one country to the other. The therapist, too, may have once been a "wandering Jew" (as were the authors of this book). Some people with such a transient personality may not really feel at home anywhere, and while they may have hoped that in Israel this basic feeling will change, the change may not be complete. This is one of the basic problems of the relationship between "I" and "We," between the individual and society in Israel. This feeling of not quite belonging, while common to immigrants from many countries, may be especially prominent among children and grandchildren of Holocaust survivors (second and third generation). Another very important aspect of this group of children of survivors involves the enormous pressure to continue the "chain of generations," which means having children. Most adults have a home, a family, and children. But one of the patients, whose story is told in this book, has not (yet?) succeeded in creating a family. Most people have a sense of belonging (to their family and to other groups), and we usually belong to a chain of generations that has not ceased. Yet there are exceptions, people who do not have this basic feeling of belongingness and continuity.

The therapist must be careful not to superimpose his/her values, identifications and belongings on the patient.

As in many other cases, one has to find the proper distance, of closeness and understanding, without causing a feeling of suffocation, to allow the patient the possibility of developing his/her autonomy, in a caring and helping atmosphere.

To be (or not to be) judgmental (Narrative 3 in contradiction to 4)

In psychotherapy one has generally to be "neutral" and nonjudgmental. But in extraordinary cases, usually when facing dilemmas, we almost have no choice but to be judgmental, to have a specific opinion about a certain issue. In such cases we must take full responsibility for our decision and our position, a position that is often educational or moral. For example, can we prescribe medication to repress the uncontrolled sexual drive of an old demented man, who demanded to have sexual intercourse with his wife, in an often unbearable way and frequency? The doctor's dilemma is: is this man insane, and should he be hospitalized? Or, is sexual intercourse one of the last pleasures that this old man still has and of which he should not be deprived? This is a dilemma, for which no right answer exists.

Prescribing medication to a demented person when the patient does not understand the reason for taking the pills is also a dilemma. Why do this, and for what purpose? Is there a "good" and "right" answer? After making such a decision, based on conviction and belief, the therapist often remains anxious and with many ethical questions unanswered. In such cases we have to take a position, and stand behind it. One cannot roll the ball to the patient's court and let patient and family decide. In such situations it is also not fair to hide behind formal regulations, or to find other ways of escape. These are situations in which we have to come out honestly with our opinion, beliefs, and conviction.

When the patient is not sane, an ethical consideration may be the following: the patient cannot judge the situation any more and is unable to decide, so the physician can decide instead of him, as if the physician were his officially appointed custodian. When the patient is sane and still in a position to decide, the therapist can advise him and pronounce clearly and honestly his/her opinion and belief. Usually a psychotherapist should remain nonjudgmental, but there are times when one must try to stop a patient's dangerous behaviors and tendencies, like a desire to take extreme risks, including in the area of sexuality.

Erotic feelings (Narratives 4, 5 and also 6)

One has to distinguish between the pleasure from sexual relationships, which are strongly prohibited in the professional context, and the pleasure of having a good and close (and even loving) relationship with a patient, which at times may be accompanied by an undeniable erotic aspect. We should accept that this dimension is part of a close relationship and friendship between two human beings. One should control and regulate this process, so that it will be helpful for the patient, and will not complicate or even destroy the relationship.

We should also be aware of behaviors, interactions, and intentions that are initiated only because the therapist enjoys them – for example, too many examinations (including touching the patient's body) or too many home visits, just because one wants to meet the patient. One should not discuss irrelevant intimate and sexual issues, just because one enjoys being a part of these intimate secrets. The aim of the doctor–patient encounter is always to treat, to care and to help patients and one is of course happy when this help has been successful.

A patient sometimes has chosen a physician (or another therapist) to discuss intimate issues. Here the patient may see the therapist as a kind of "parent" to whom he/she can talk safely and in utmost confidentiality. It is natural that one listens to such secrets with a caring attitude and a professional ear.

A new perspective (Narratives 6 and 15)

Especially in cases in which one feels stuck, or in cases in which a negative attitude towards the patient has developed, it is advisable to change the setting or to broaden the area. One way of doing this is to ask patients to tell their biography, their life history. This gives therapists a better understanding of the patients' background and enables therapists to gain a new perspective. One can also change the form and setting of treatment, or the combination of people in the office, e.g. to ask a patient whom we have seen individually to come with his or her spouse. Our objective, as therapists, is that during the process of treatment we always see a new and changing horizon. It is very important to invent new therapeutic interventions, to be creative and to look for new perspectives – for example, the salutogenetic attitude that asks: why and how does a person remain relatively healthy? What were the inner and outer resources that this person could mobilize? How to find a novel way for caring for a patient psychotherapeutically, without talking (Narrative 16)?

Guilt and guilt feelings (Narrative 6)

Martin Buber differentiates between guilt and guilt feelings. "Guilt," or being guilty, is in the domain of law, the police, the court, and the ethical committees of professional organizations. "Guilt feelings" are human feelings, connected with ethics, conscience, one's subjective feeling of responsibility, and one's active or passive part in the fate of another. There is a certain connection between guilt feelings and compassion – for example, when we kill a person who suddenly crossed a road at a forbidden place. Nobody blamed us, the police said that we acted well and that it was not our fault, and the insurance company has not sued us. Yet, in spite of all that, we feel that we killed a person, perhaps because we reacted too slowly.

Buber writes that if we do not have guilt feelings in such a situation, we would not be human beings. It is human to have guilt feelings, even when one is not guilty. Physicians and other therapists often have such experiences. A physician acted reasonably yet the patient deteriorated, or even died. The patient, or the family, may be angry with the physician. We are not guilty in the eyes of the law, but our human condition creates feelings of guilt.

Different agendas (Narrative 6)

Sometimes the therapist and the patient have different agendas. They may even have different basic goals.

There is also a possibility that on a certain day the therapist is preoccupied by his/her inner world, memories, past experiences, or special national events, while at the same time, the patient is involved in his/her personal issues. In such a situation a distance may be created, which might turn the words of the patient to something not relevant for the therapist and vice versa. The patient here may be perceived as not being interesting and boring, compared to those things which occupy the therapist's mind.

It is important to become aware of this situation and to try to bring the therapeutic process and the doctor–patient relationship back to the main road, where the focus is always on the patient.

The dying patient (Narratives 7, 14 and 17)

Sometimes patients confess to their physicians, close to their death, a personal story, often a secret and complicated story, one that they had never told anybody. Like confession before a clergyman, they put this memory in the hands (and head and heart) of the physician for safekeeping.

It may be a horrible story, like things that happened during the Holocaust. Sometimes one is frightened to listen to these narratives, and the fact that the patient has chosen us, and we are the only ones who have to hear it, evokes in us much anxiety. Talking with a person who is about to die may be sad and frightening. It may cause anxiety, as the therapist is helpless and not able to help any more; our role of being a physician has ended. This situation may remind us of our own death. At the very same time, the physician may have a feeling of satisfaction and dignity.

As physicians, we might be proud that the patient has chosen us as someone whom he or she is able to trust. We might be proud that we were chosen to hear a story that will be kept in our memory, when the patient has passed on.

It is important to assist dying people to die in their own style. We clinicians may experience a deep sense of satisfaction and grief, when we have the opportunity and the duty to be with a dying patient whom we have loved and cared for over a long time (Narrative 17). In the relationship with a dying patient, the physician ceases to be a "savior" and healer, and is then much more a caring person who accompanies the dying patient on his/her final journey.

Caring for patients and fatalism (Narrative 8)

At times, therapists play different roles. Mostly, they *do* – they are healers, professionals who have to act, to do something, to save. But sometimes they just have to *be* – to be with the patient, to support, to care, to make things easier. By "being with," one might give the patient something that is very important even though one might think that "I have not done anything." There are patients, families, societies, and cultures that perceive disease as fate. This fatalism might be seen as negative, depressive, with much guilt feelings, appraising the disease as a punishment perhaps, like Job's lot, an unjustified and undeserved punishment.

But fatalism may be positive: "Let us wait and see, let us hope, a miracle might happen, I may be lucky. Let things develop." (Sometimes a medical prognosis might just be wrong.)

However, it should be pointed out that fatalism can be mixed with passivity, which might be harmful. Passivity may appear together with "secondary gain," meaning that the patient is quite happy being a chronically ill person, or an invalid with all the economical, psychological, and social gains. Conversely, fatalism may be associated with acceptance and hope.

The symptom (Narratives 8 and 9)

Symptoms, especially functional ones, often have a meaning, and body language can express distress, conflicts, desires, etc., in severe cases when anger cannot be verbalized. Many times it is impossible to speak about these feelings, or it may be too dangerous and forbidden to do so and even to express them nonverbally by shouting or crying. When a certain situation in life causes, for example, the feeling "of a lump in one's throat" that may explode at any moment, the patient has to swallow these feelings, when suddenly symptoms such as reflux, gastric pain, or heartburn may develop. These symptoms may be connected with the described stress.

A psychotherapist may reach out together with the patient, and find ways in which these feelings can be expressed and articulated in words. Such verbalizing may be possible, at first, only in the office, but later, in a controlled and refined (sublimated) way, also outside the therapeutic relationship, and then the symptom may disappear. As a psychotherapist one often needs to observe a patient over time, to be a good listener, until reaching that suitable moment, in a regulated way, when one is able to discuss with the patient the distress that he/she "has swallowed."

Relations with a second therapist (Narrative 11)

Sometimes a patient is in parallel treatment with two therapists, as when being treated by a clinical psychologist and a family physician. Difficulties and frictions may develop between the two therapists, if, for example, the family physician feels he/she is being manipulated. Such a situation may arise if a psychotherapist (clinical psychologist) who had never contacted the family physician about a common patient suddenly phones with information.

The astonished family physician is happy at first, but then realizes that the psychotherapist just tried to use him, as he told him on the phone that their common patient disappeared from psychotherapy, and has not paid. The physician first feels responsibility and guilt, and next understands that he has been manipulated. Indeed, it is possible that the physician is being exploited and activated by the psychotherapist, but the patient might also be manipulating both therapists.

In another case, a patient may tell the family physician that the psychotherapist, with whom the patient is also in treatment, has told him to stop a certain medication, as it interferes with the process of psychotherapy. The physician becomes very angry with the psychotherapist for telling him what to do. Afterwards it turns out that the therapist had never given this advice and that the patient "misunderstood" him. Both clinicians may have been manipulated by the patient in this case. In such cases important issues of boundaries and limits of responsibilities arise. The clinician may have this internal dialogue: "How can I keep my autonomy as a family physician? How can I make clear boundaries and contracts, avoiding a conflict with the other therapist yet without becoming too paternalistic towards the patient?".

Payment and reward (Narrative 11)

Therapists and physicians in the public service are used to treating patients who have pre-paid for their treatment and who do not pay them directly. However, in private practice, the patient pays the therapist directly, sometimes with an efficient secretary as intermediary.

Some physicians and other therapists find it difficult to ask to be paid and to receive money. It is just these professionals who must be aware of the need to keep payments coming regularly and on schedule, without deviating from agreed-upon conditions. This might be difficult when a patient is in a continued and long relationship with us, as in psychotherapy. It becomes even more difficult when the patient is a very nice person that we love, or whom we pity. One has always to keep in mind that an hour of therapy costs money. When one does not insist on this rule, the treatment is in great danger of entering emotional confusion, often with projective identifications including blaming and guilt feelings. This is a situation that is certainly not healthy, neither for the patient nor for the therapist. It should be a golden rule, that nonpsychotic and adult patients must take the responsibility for their steps and decisions and for their consequences – and for their payments.

The child within us (Narrative 12)

There are adult, and even old, patients who behave like children. They may seek a "parent" in a physician or therapist, even when the professional is much younger than the patient. Similarly, within us therapists, there is always a hidden, sometimes very sensitive, child.

The same cultural background and language (Narrative 13)

Having a doctor–patient or psychotherapeutic relationship with a patient born in the same country of origin, coming from a similar socio-cultural background and having the same mother tongue, facilitates the creation of good communication. But, such closeness may also be "dangerous" and an opening for talk that becomes gossip or too personal. As in all settings, in this case too, one has to endeavor to keep the boundaries and limits of professional treatment, and not fall into the trap of familiarity.

Life cycle and chain of generations (Narrative 18)

With this last reflection I will close my comments. Therapists may be the witness of very important processes of human development. I refer to the process of growing, becoming mature, becoming old and declining in one's facilities, until death. The therapist may be a witness to a multigenerational process, of a new generation coming after a previous one, a chain that will hopefully never cease. As therapists, we ourselves pass through all these stages in the life cycle, and it is fascinating and moving to observe the process, as patients share their journeys with us.

Index